Susan H. Johnston, M.S.W.
Deborah A. Kraut, M.I.L.R.

*

PREGNANCY
BEDREST

*

A Guide for the Pregnant Woman and Her Family

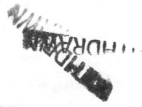

AN OWL BOOK
HENRY HOLT AND COMPANY
New York

Henry Holt and Company, Inc.
Publishers since 1866
115 West 18th Street
New York, New York 10011

Henry Holt® is a registered trademark
of Henry Holt and Company, Inc.

Library of Congress Cataloging-in-Publication Data
Johnston, Susan H.
Pregnancy bedrest: a guide for the pregnant woman and her family/
Susan H. Johnston and Deborah A. Kraut.—1st ed.
p. cm.
"An Owl book."
Includes Index.
1. Pregnancy.   2. Pregnancy, Complications of—Prevention.
3. Bedrest—Psychological aspects.   4. Pregnant women—
Family relationships.   I. Kraut, Deborah A. II. Title.
RG525.J64 1990   90-36263
618.3—dc20   CIP
ISBN 0-8050-1350-4

First Owl Book Edition—1990

Designed by Kathryn Parise

All first editions are printed on acid-free paper.∞

7 9 10 8 6

Portions of this book were privately published in the booklet *Pregnancy
Bedrest: A Guidebook for the Pregnant Woman and Her Family.*

To
our mothers and fathers
and
our husbands, Rick and Alan,
and
our children, Kylie, Ryan,
and Julia Rose

CONTENTS

✳

YOUR MEDICAL MANAGEMENT TEAM
59

TEMPORARILY REORGANIZING YOUR LIFE
75

BEDREST AWAY FROM HOME
117

TAKING STOCK OF ALL THE CHANGES
137

FOREWORD

＊

Pregnancy bedrest is a tried-and-true remedy, used throughout the ages to improve a high-risk mother's chances of delivering a healthy baby. New understanding about fetal growth and development and about the causes of hypertension and preterm labor, has led to a greater appreciation of the benefits of bedrest for some pregnant women. But despite these well-documented benefits, as you have probably learned, pregnancy bedrest can be *very* stressful.

If pregnancy bedrest is recommended for you, undoubtedly you are concerned about yourself and your baby . . . and you may be wondering how you are going to manage all of your usual responsibilities. *Pregnancy Bedrest: A Guide for the Pregnant Woman and Her Family* is a wonderfully thorough reference that will help make your days of confinement a little more comfortable, a little less inconvenient, and a lot more manageable. Use this book as a travelogue to find the information you need to make this "high-risk" journey to the birth of your baby a little easier.

If you feel you don't have much control over this journey to birth, you are not alone. But *Pregnancy Bedrest* will help you understand that, indeed, you *do* have choices over how you will spend the next days or weeks. This book will give you tips for managing day-to-day inconveniences and dilemmas, such as how to keep from spilling crumbs in your bed, how to keep the house clean, and how to care for your other children. But even more important, it will coach you on how to turn this period of bedrest into an opportunity for personal growth.

All pregnant women want information that will help them make informed decisions for themselves and for their babies. I know you will find the practical information in *Pregnancy Bedrest* helpful to you as you face the challenge of therapeutic bedrest. I wish a safe journey to delivery to both you and your baby. This book will surely help you on that journey.

Rae K. Grad, R.N., Ph.D.
Executive Director
National Commission to Prevent Infant Mortality

FOREWORD

✳

You have been given a very difficult decision. You have been told that you must spend more time in bed to improve the chances of the health and even the survival of your baby or babies. Hopefully you obtained enough information from your health-care providers so that you understand the reason(s) for your increased risk of having a complication and the rationale behind the recommendation of bedrest. Now comes the hard part, carrying out your decision to stay in bed for your health and/or the health of your baby (or babies).

Pregnancy Bedrest: A Guide for the Pregnant Woman and Her Family is an outstanding tour through the emotions, the risks, the reasons, and the coping that accompany a bedrest pregnancy. Though nothing will help you more than your partner and your knowledge that you are doing the right thing, this book comes in a close third. It is sensitive to your thoughts and emotions; after all, it was written by two bedresters! It is medically accurate in the few places it is necessary to discuss medical concepts. It is also sensitive to your budget. The ideas that have associated costs are identified, and alternatives are suggested if possible. Most important, it was written with humor and love. Though the love must come from that which the authors gave and give to their children, and that which they give to their clients, there is plenty more in the pages of this well-written book. Use it, enjoy it, and share it. It is certainly the only medically related book I've ever read that brought tears to my eyes!

David A. Nagey, M.D., Ph.D.
Associate Professor
Director, Division of Maternal Fetal Medicine
Department of Obstetrics and Gynecology
University of Maryland School of Medicine

INTRODUCTION

*

If you are pregnant and reading this book, you've begun dealing with one of the most terrifying experiences a woman can have. You have been told by your doctor that your pregnancy has developed a medical complication: you've heard the words "at risk."

Your doctor gave you a name for your specific complication and then may have continued talking about a medication you would be taking, possible surgery, and immediate restricted activity, *including bedrest.*

Suddenly, your world seemed to have shattered. You tried to stay calm and listen to what your doctor was telling you, but you were also thinking about your baby, the father, your children, your job, his job, money, parents, cooking, cleaning, eating, shopping, the holidays, lying in a bed all day—alone.

You were probably almost frozen in shock.

The worst has happened: your pregnancy has been threatened with a medical problem. While you're trying to understand what has happened, you are told to stop your activities, give up all that you do, and remain in bed.

Our pregnancies were at-risk and required bedrest, too. We wrote this book to share with you ways to get through each day of a medically complicated pregnancy requiring restricted activity. These are not just our own ideas, but the ideas and stories of many pregnancy bedresters and their families. This book has practical advice, checklists, how-tos, reassurance for your feelings, and even some bedrest humor.

Please remember that this book is not intended to give medical advice or be a substitute for proper medical care. Whenever you have a question or a problem concerning your medical condition, talk to your doctor or your nurse.

Although it is often assumed that there is a man around the house, we realize that this is not the case for many women, including those on bedrest. So we decided to simplify matters by calling men in this book "fathers" or "partners."

Read this book any way you want to, in any order. Start with what you need to know first, and don't force yourself to read any chapter that upsets you! We know one woman who simply held this book next to her for a few days.

Reread chapters as your pregnancy progresses: ideas that didn't make sense one week will be exactly what you need a week or two later. Share this book with your family so that they can help you deal with your bedrest routine.

*

GETTING
THE NEWS

*

1

✳

How a Bedrest
Pregnancy Begins

There are three ways in which a pregnancy becomes a bedrest pregnancy. All three begin with a doctor-patient talk. You may have gone to the office for one of your regular checkups, or you were seeing your doctor today because you experienced a warning signal you read about in a pamphlet, or you wanted to see your doctor ahead of schedule because you were experiencing the same feelings you had when a previous pregnancy "went sour."

Then, during the preparations for your physical examination, the medical staff seemed a little different. Instead of waiting with the other pregnant women, you may have been taken to an exam room as soon as you walked in the door. After the nurse took your vital signs, she seemed a little quiet. During your examination, your doctor was suddenly "all business" and was signaling to the nurse while closing the door to your exam room. You could almost feel the difference in the air when you sat down to talk a few minutes later.

What follows are three versions of the beginning of pregnancy bedrest:

SCENE ONE

DOCTOR: Well, Ms. Smith, we've talked about the possibility of this pregnancy developing a complication. . . .
(Pick *a*, *b*, c, or *d*):

a. Your previous pregnancy . . . blurp, geek, fizz . . .
b. Your mother's pregnancy . . . fizz, buzz, buzz . . .
c. Your preexisting medical condition . . . buzz, tweep
d. Your history of infertility might . . . buzz buzz
   I've found that _____ in my examination, and you
   need to buzz, blurp, geek, BEDREST, home, hospital,
   buzz, buzz, immediately, Ms. Smith. . . .

Ms. SMITH (*very pale, shaking*): Doctor, could you repeat what you said?

SCENE TWO

DOCTOR: Well, Ms. Smith, I'm glad you telephoned to come to see me today, because you have developed a _____ complication . . . buzz buzz, usually seen in one of the warning signals . . . buzz, buzz, blurp, geek, BEDREST, buzz, buzz, home, hospital, buzz, buzz, immediately, Ms. Smith. . . .

Ms. SMITH (*very pale, shaking*): Could you repeat that, please?

SCENE THREE

DOCTOR: Well, Ms. Smith, sometimes even the most normal pregnancy can develop a . . . buzz, buzz, _____ complication, fortunately . . . time buzz, buzz, BEDREST . . . hospital . . . call buzz buzz, home . . . new techniques, blurb, geek . . .

Ms. SMITH (*very pale, shaking*): I didn't understand. Could you say that again?

AND ANOTHER SCENE THAT SOMETIMES OCCURS

DOCTOR: Well, Ms. Smith, I know you're happy about having a multiple gestation . . . buzz, buzz, perfectly . . . might need to . . . BEDREST . . . he must be . . . buzz blurb . . . rest . . . close monitoring. . . .

MS. SMITH (*very pale, shaking*): Doctor, what do you mean, "multiple"?

So the three beginnings to a medically complicated pregnancy that requires bedrest are:

1. Your medical history, including previous pregnancies, and/or your family medical history indicates to your doctor that you might develop a medical problem during this pregnancy.
2. You read about the warning signals in a pregnancy and you experience one of these signals.
3. You have no history of medical problems, no family history of medical problems, and experience no symptoms. Your doctor discovers your medical complication during a routine checkup.

Some of the pregnancy complications that are commonly aided by bedrest positioning include: high blood pressure (pregnancy-induced hypertension, preeclampsia, eclampsia), vaginal bleeding (placenta previa, abruptio placentae), premature labor, and a change in the condition of the cervix (incompetent cervix, cervical effacement). Less common complications, such as varicose veins, may benefit from special positioning.

If a previous pregnancy resulted in a fetal loss, stillbirth, or premature baby, the next pregnancy receives closer monitoring and may require bedrest, too.

A pregnancy that is a multiple gestation, that is, two or more developing fetuses, automatically requires closer medical monitoring. When related medical conditions develop, a multiple gestation may become a bedrest pregnancy.

It's perfectly normal to listen to the first few words your doctor says and then be unable to understand or focus on the following sentences. Sometimes the news is so difficult and painful to hear that you shut out part of it to protect yourself. In the first few minutes, you may find yourself feeling anger, fear, and a sadness as though you had lost this baby.

What you have lost is your idea of a normal pregnancy. You had made plans, reserved your place in childbirth classes: you had an image of yourself very pregnant, happily leading an active life in preparation for the birth of your baby.

Now your doctor has advised you to go home to bed. The last thing you want to do at this minute is go home and lie down on your bed! So, like the fictional Ms. Smith, you ask your doctor to repeat his or her words, all the while thinking, "Why bedrest for my pregnancy?"

2

＊

Why Bedrest for
My Pregnancy?

Your doctor has prescribed restricted activities for you, including periods of time during which you remain lying down in a specific position. The easiest place to lie down is your bed, and that's why your doctor says "bedrest."

You have one or more medical conditions that may stabilize, that is, remain the same, or at least not get any worse if you begin bedrest. Some medical conditions may actually improve with prescribed bedrest positioning during a pregnancy. Your doctor and nurse will explain to you the specific nature of your medical complication and how bedrest can aid in its stabilization or improvement. What works for one pregnancy will work differently for another. Each bedrest situation is unique.

It is important to understand that you are not just getting into bed to sleep or to "take it easy." You are not starting bedrest to recover or to "get well." You are not now "sick."

Prescribed bedrest positioning is active work for you. Once you have positioned yourself correctly, you have to think about what you do all day and learn to accomplish these tasks while maintaining this position.

We often wish doctors would write "pregnancy bedrest positioning" on a prescription slip, just like any other prescribed medication in the management of your pregnancy. When you have been
prescribed pregnancy bedrest, you are working to achieve two
goals for the medical management of your pregnancy:

1. to maintain your body in a position that does the most good
for your developing pregnancy.

2. to minimize all other physical activities that can put stress on
your specific medical complication.

The hidden medicine in pregnancy bedrest is *gravity*. The
earth's gravity pulls on different parts of your body when you are
lying down from when you are standing up. By positioning your
body in a specific way, gravity can aid in stabilizing or even improv-
ing your medical condition.

Oh, come on, you're thinking, *this is too easy an answer.* Your
doctor and nurse can explain the details of how your body functions
lying down during your pregnancy. They can tell you how lying
down quietly calms your uterus. They can explain to you how lying
down on your left side changes the blood flow to your uterus and
how this change affects your medical condition. They can also
explain how elevating your hips above your shoulders is effective
for gravity-sensitive medical complications.

You can "rest assured" that pregnancy bedrest positioning has a
positive medical history for certain medical complications.

Why can't I just take medication instead? The answer to this
question is that your doctor may prescribe medication for you and
you may have surgery, too. Pregnancy bedrest is part of a variety of
medical treatments, each accomplishing a slightly different purpose.

What if I just don't want to get into bed? Don't ignore your
doctor's advice. Instead, talk frankly to your doctor about your
concerns. Learn specifically why your doctor is advising a period of
lying down during your pregnancy. Make sure you understand the
restrictions in your life you are advised to make.

If you do not want to start bedrest, understand the pros and
cons of unrestricted activities and the possible outcome for your
pregnancy if you continue your activities without bedrest.

How many pregnant women need bedrest? We don't know. Doctors are not required to report statistics on how many patients are advised to restrict their activities, including periods of bedrest. Likewise, they are not required to report statistics on exactly how many patients develop specific complications during their pregnancies.

Every pregnant woman on bedrest starts as a statistic of "one." But just because there are no accurate statistics about bedrest, this does not mean that no one else is going through pregnancy with restricted activities. Pregnancy bedresters can't have parades. We can't meet each other in the supermarket or the aerobics class and chat. We meet each other in the doctor's office or while waiting for a medical test or because we learn about each other and telephone to talk. That's how we, the authors, met.

When does a pregnant woman usually begin bedrest? There are great variations in the point in your pregnancy at which you begin therapeutic bedrest and in how long this bedrest period will be. Some women have been advised to start their bedrest at the beginning of their pregnancies, others will start during the second trimester, while still others will start bedrest during the last part of their pregnancies and remain on bedrest until their babies are born. One of the authors "lucked out" and got to spend all three trimesters on bedrest!

Your doctor may prescribe pregnancy bedrest in "gradual doses," increasing or decreasing your activities during your pregnancy. Or you may be started at "full-strength," stopping all activities for the rest of your pregnancy.

My doctor talks about "weeks of bedrest." How does that match the trimesters of a pregnancy? Pregnancy bedrest changes the way you date and count the duration of your pregnancy.

When you first became pregnant, your doctor took the date your last menstrual period began, added 280 days, and gave you a due date for the birth of your baby. The number of 280 is equal to ten lunar months of 28 days. You completed the first lunar month by the time you missed your menstrual period and began to think you were pregnant. The remaining nine lunar months are traditionally thought of as three trimesters.

Pregnancy bedrest is usually stated in weeks. Your doctor tells you that bedrest will be for so many weeks, or until the xth week of your pregnancy. You will need frequent appointments. Certain weeks in your bedrest pregnancy take on a new meaning: weeks during which certain problems can occur, weeks when you must start or can stop medication, and weeks that are used for estimates of the size and development of your baby.

It's a good idea for you to think about your bedrest pregnancy in terms of weeks rather than trimesters. A trimester is an impossibly long time to think about when being advised to start bedrest. Thinking in terms of weeks, even days, enables you to manage your bedrest as a series of short-term goals. When you concentrate on getting through one week, you set a goal you can reach within just seven days. Yes, a bedrest pregnancy is a game of numbers—tricks you play with counting to help you feel you are accomplishing something for your baby while you are lying in bed. Just remember that each day you successfully manage on bedrest really does count.

3

*

Immediate Arrangements

During each of my four pregnancies, one office visit always resulted in admission to the hospital. You'd think by the third time, certainly by the fourth, I'd know what to do and who to call. But I always collapsed. Thank goodness the office staff had enough "practice" with me to know how to get in touch with my family and even who to call at my job.

When a pregnancy becomes high-risk, medical treatment to save it can be swift. A woman may need to be hospitalized immediately for surgery and for medication therapies. Full-strength bedrest positioning may be tried first in a hospital setting to determine whether therapeutic positioning can be effective in stabilizing a medical complication.

Swift medical treatment may also be started at home. A doctor may prescribe immediate bedrest, advising a woman literally to go home and go to bed.

If you've just been told by your doctor that you need to start pregnancy bedrest immediately and you were fortunate enough to

11

have also been given this book, this chapter will help you organize your thoughts right now.

If you are reading this book several days after starting on a low-dose or full-strength bedrest positioning plan, this chapter can help you develop a strategy for the future. As you develop your strategy, be sure to update your patient chart for who to contact in an emergency.

First, find a quiet room in your doctor's office where you can sit and make telephone calls. If there are no examination rooms with phones, ask to use a vacant doctor's office. You need to call people and you may need to wait for calls back to you. Take as much time as you need and don't worry about upsetting the office routine—the staff understands your situation.

Make sure that each person you telephone knows whether you are being admitted to a hospital or going home. Write down the name and telephone number of your doctor's office and the name of the hospital if you are being admitted. Keep these numbers in front of you as you talk so you can "read" them to each person. Several situations that may apply to you are described below.

Your Baby's Father

If he is right there in the doctor's office, recognize that he, too, has just heard that your pregnancy is high-risk. He may be experiencing some moments of frozen shock, too. He will drive you home or to the hospital. He may then get back behind the wheel and begin driving around trying to do all the impossible tasks of getting you started on bedrest. Make sure he is calm enough to start driving.

If he is at work right now, time is the most important issue in figuring out where to meet. If he is only a few minutes away, he may be able to come to the doctor's office and be with you. If his location is more than a half-hour's drive, it may be better to meet at home or at the hospital.

He may also be the "emergency phone contact" for your job, for your other child at school, and for your doctor's office. It may make more sense for him to handle child-care arrangements and other telephone work before he travels to you.

There are no rules for couples handling crises. You do what makes the most sense right now for your own situation.

"How Do I Get Where I Am Supposed to Be Going?"

You may not be allowed to drive yourself to your destination. Let the office staff arrange transportation to the hospital or to your home. They know the most reliable taxi service to use and the doctor's office may be a familiar address to taxi drivers.

You Are Currently Working

If you had planned to return to your job after this appointment, you need to call your workplace. If you feel you can make the telephone call yourself, call your supervisor and explain that you have a medical complication that requires immediate medical treatment. If you don't feel emotionally ready to do it yourself, ask your doctor's secretary or your nurse to make this telephone call for you. Neither will explain all the personal details of your pregnancy, but will make sure that your supervisor understands that you have a serious medical problem.

Remember that the people in your workplace should know where you are going after you leave your doctor's office. If you are unable to reach your baby's father, he may try to contact you later today at your job. If you are unable to reach your family, they will call your coworkers if you are not home at your usual time. Family and friends know where you work—they rarely know the phone number of your doctor.

You Have a Baby-sitter at Home with Your Other Child

If a baby-sitter is watching your child in your home, plan for that person to remain in charge until a family member or friend can arrive. Find out how long your sitter can extend her work hours. Then, phone a family member or friend to come directly to your home. Make sure to call your sitter *again* to tell her the name of this person and the time she will arrive.

If you are coming home to bedrest, tell your sitter when she can expect you. She can help you get from your doorway to your bedroom without tripping over toys and getting sidetracked by a crying child. Although you are home, your sitter should remain in charge of your child until your friend or family member arrives. Even if you are not feeling any physical discomfort, the office visit will have emotionally exhausted you. You may really want to lie down and gather back your strength rather than start playing with your child or preparing supper.

If you are being admitted to the hospital, make sure your baby-sitter knows the name of the hospital.

You may be tempted to talk briefly to a young child, but if you are very upset, your voice will carry your fears and your child may begin to cry and ask you questions. Then, you'll begin to cry, too. It's better to concentrate on your young child's safety and care now and talk directly to him or her when you are calmer.

Your Other Child Is in School

You need to arrange for the care of your child from the time school is dismissed until the father or a family member can arrive. Try to keep your child's scheduled day as normal as possible.

Does your child play at the home of a friend right after school? Can you call that child's mother now? If you answered yes twice, you can solve this afterschool problem quickly. Be sure that this mother knows if you are going home or to a hospital.

Maybe you can't remember the phone numbers of any child's mother. Or you can't get in touch with a mother. You need to call the school office. Explain your current situation briefly and ask them to help locate the mothers who could help you.

If the school staff is unable to contact a mother you know, they need to contact the "emergency person" listed on your child's school records for emergencies. That may be your baby's father.

Remember that school offices remain open after dismissal time. Your child can remain in the school office until the father, a family member, or a friend can come. If the person who will pick up your child is not listed in the school records, make sure the school staff knows the name of this person.

It is best for you and your school-age child to talk about this immediate arrangement. He can be paged from his class to the school office to talk to you. Even if you are very upset and your voice carries your fears, a school-age child will be reassured by listening to your instructions. He will understand that you have a problem, you are handling it, and you are continuing to care for him.

Make sure the school staff knows where you are going after the doctor's office. They need to know the name of the hospital if you are being hospitalized.

Your Other Child Attends an Afterschool Program

Who picks up your child at the end of the program? Is another parent authorized to pick up your child from this program? If you answered yes twice, you use this arrangement.

As above, if you can't get in touch with this parent, the program staff need to contact the "emergency person" listed in your child's records. Bingo—your baby's father again! As above, you may need to contact another person to pick up your child and you should let the program staff know the name of this person.

You Were Supposed to Take Care of Other School-Age Children This Afternoon

What did you do when you were supposed to "take the kids" and you got sick? If you and the other mothers have ever had to rearrange the child care prior to today, you know what calls to make now. If you are not able to get in touch with one of the mothers, it is important enough to contact the school office and ask the staff to get in touch with the parent of that child.

You Were in Charge of a Church/Civic/Social Event This Evening

Your family knew you were going to do this activity. Don't worry. They will get in touch with the right people. The members of the program group have had to deal with illnesses and will know what to do.

You Are Feeling Too Upset or Ill to Make Telephone Calls

Let your nurse or the secretary telephone your workplace and make calls to the school and the baby-sitter. You filled out a form stating who your doctor should contact in case of an emergency: the office staff will contact this person and begin to coordinate the telephone calls.

Don't worry. This office staff deals every day with maternity patients who are headed for the hospital for routine and nonroutine reasons. They are experienced in helping women make quick re-arrangements of their schedules!

You Have Too Many Telephone Calls to Make

See above. Ask the office staff to help you make calls.

Your Car Is Stranded and the Traffic Meter Has Expired

Your family and friends will handle "travel arrangements" for your car, probably by late evening. If your car was ticketed, check off the portion requesting a court date to appeal the violation. Write on this ticket that you are temporarily disabled and will need to arrange a court date for when your doctor states you can travel.

You Made All the Calls and Arrangements, But You Don't Know How You'll Manage the Next Weeks

Remember in the book, *Gone with the Wind*, what Scarlett O'Hara said when faced with a problem that had no immediate answer: "I'll worry about that tomorrow. After all, tomorrow is another day."

Tomorrow, after you've managed the first hours of bedrest, you will be able to think more clearly and find the answers to many of these questions.

*

THE NUTS
AND BOLTS
OF BEDREST

*

4

*

Physical Positions

Throughout each day, you will be either lying down or sitting up or standing. Every high-risk pregnant woman will spend some time in each of these physical positions each day. How *much* time you are allowed to spend lying down, sitting up, or standing, depends on your specific medical condition. As your pregnancy progresses, the amount of time spent in each position will vary.

Lying Down

Let's begin with the different basic positions for lying down. Usually, you will be lying down on your side. You may be told to lie only on your left side, or you may be allowed to alternate between lying on your left side and your right side.

There are two ways you can lie on your side:

1. Lying completely on one side so that one of your shoulders and the mattress form the shape of the capital letter *L*. One shoulder will point straight up to the ceiling in this position. See figure 1.

2. Lying on one side so that your shoulders and the mattress form the shape of the letter V. Your shoulders will be pointed at an angle toward one wall in this position. See figure 2.

When you are lying on your side in either position, you'll find that it is easier to view a television set that is at the side of your bed. See figure 1.

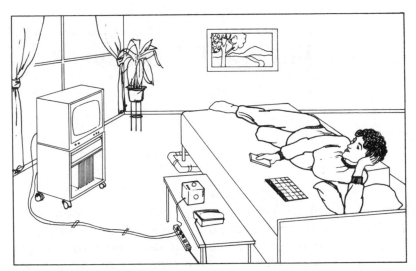

Fig. 1

Lying Down and Raising Your Hips

For certain medical conditions, your therapeutic position will also include raising your hips so that they are higher than your shoulders. The first time this position is described by your doctor or your nurse, you might picture yourself lying head down on a playground sliding board, gripping onto the edges to keep from crashing to the ground. But the elevation or tilt of your hips is just a few inches. See figure 1 above and figure 2 on the following page. You won't feel very uncomfortable, but neither will you feel totally relaxed. The best way to cope with the tilt position is to accept that it is a constant annoyance.

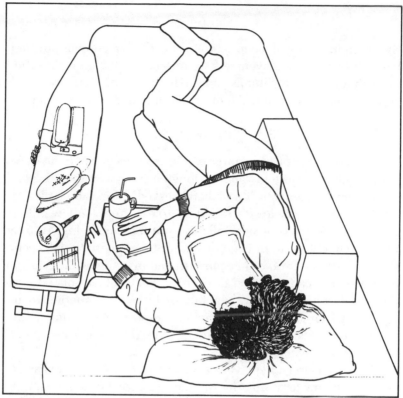

Fig. 2

The one way that you will *not* be positioned is lying flat on your
back. You may notice that lying on your back makes you uncomfortable. That is because the weight of your uterus by mid-pregnancy
(or sooner, with a multiple gestation) presses on the major blood
vessels in your abdomen. The pressing on the blood vessels
changes your blood pressure and the blood flow to your uterus.
Your feelings of discomfort are Mother Nature's way of telling you
to roll over to your side!

There will be times when you feel the urge to lie flat and stretch
to uncramp your back. You may be given a few exercises to help
ease the tension of one physical position. But you won't be sleeping
or lying on your back for long periods of time.

Sleeping

Every night, you will sleep in your specific lying-down position. It's not easy to force yourself to remain in the same position throughout the night. But as you gradually develop a daily schedule of things to do, you will feel tired enough at night to sleep.

Sitting Up

When your doctor or your nurse explained the correct lying-down position for you and told you how long each day you should spend lying down, you probably immediately asked, "What about meals?"

It's not necessary to sit straight up to eat a meal. A few pillows placed underneath your side will raise you sufficiently higher to eat a sandwich, cut meat, or even drink hot tea. Digestion will occur, even on a tilt, and you can become skilled in eating while lying on your side. But eating in bed is a chore. You can feel isolated from your family when you hear them talking together in another room. So requests for sitting-up meal privileges are very common, and some accommodation can be made, provided the pregnancy medical condition *remains* stable.

When you are lying on your side or on a tilt, you really have to think about how to sit up. The woman in figure 3 is demonstrating the "bedrester push-up," using both arms on the side of the bed to push herself up to a sitting position, without straining her abdominal muscles.

Once a time limit for sitting up is set, use your time wisely. For example, if you are allowed to sit up for one hour each day, you might want to use the time for one meal with your family. Or you might want to take just ten minutes to prop yourself up in bed for each meal and then sit up in your bed for a half hour to do some personal grooming.

Standing Up

Sitting up is associated with eating, and standing up is always associated with walking to your bathroom. After you asked about meals, you probably asked your doctor or your nurse, "What about

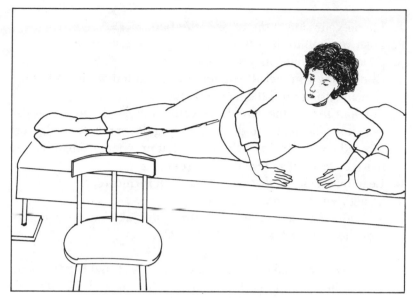

Fig. 3

going to the bathroom?" To rephrase that question, what you really wanted to know is if you could walk to the bathroom to use the toilet. And that's what bathroom privileges are: standing and walking to the toilet.

Lying down all day, with sitting-up privileges for meals and standing-up privileges for using the toilet, is the most common combination for pregnancy bedrest. Again, the combination depends upon stabilizing your medical condition during your high-risk pregnancy.

Standing up and walking is the biggest physical change from lying down. After you have spent a few days lying down, it is normal to feel a bit light-headed when you begin to stand up. You need to change your physical position slowly while placing minimal strain on your abdominal muscles.

There are eight steps to remember when you are getting out of bed. After you read these steps, look at figure 3 again and note that a sturdy piece of furniture is placed next to the bedside. If you are experiencing light-headed feelings, have someone nearby to help you, if possible.

1. Lie on your side at the edge of the bed.
2. Push yourself to the sitting-up position (see figure 3).
3. Sit still for about thirty seconds.
4. Check how you feel. If you feel light-headed while sitting up, remain sitting until the feeling fades.
5. Put your feet on the floor. Have your slippers placed so that you can slide your feet into them. Bending down to put on slippers can make you feel dizzy. Besides, what pregnant woman can see her feet, even if she isn't on bedrest?
6. Lean one hand on that sturdy piece of furniture.
7. Straighten your knees to stand.
8. Wait about thirty seconds, standing, to make sure you are not light-headed before you begin to walk.

Once you are walking, remember to walk straight to the bathroom and then straight back to your bed. Try to get back into your bed slowly, reversing the eight steps above.

Showers and Baths

See Chapter 9, "Bathroom Privileges."

Traveling to Your Doctor

Yes, in most situations, you will be sitting up, getting dressed, and traveling to your doctor's office for checkups. See Chapter 11, "Working with Your Doctor."

Balancing Your Days

You may learn that the total time you are allowed to be out of your lying-down position must include your meals, the trips to the toilet, and bathing. So, one day may become the "bath day," when you do everything in your lying-down position to save the time you need to stand up for a shower. The next day may be the "supper with the family" night. The "doctor appointment day" may require a quiet day before, with only a brief shower, and a quiet day afterward.

It takes a while to learn to balance your bedrest days. This is a completely new experience for you: pregnancy bedrest is *not* the same as recovering from surgery, lying in bed with the chicken pox, or lying on a sunny beach.

This book will help you with ideas for making the most of your bedrest positioning time and for making efficient use of your time sitting up or standing.

5

***

Basic Equipment

In the previous chapter, you learned about the basic physical positions for side-lying, tilting your hips, sitting up, and getting out of bed. Now you need to figure out how to maintain your specific bedrest position correctly and comfortably. Once you've mastered the basics, you can quickly move to setting up your room, planning your days, buying clothes, and even scheduling a haircut.

Here is a list of the absolute basics for maintaining your bedrest position. This is the equipment you need twenty-four hours a day, every day during your bedrest. If you can't afford some of these items, discuss your financial situation with your nurse or your doctor.

To begin, you have to lie on a flat surface. In your home, that's your mattress. It's flat, wide, and flexible. In most instances, your own mattress, bed frame, and several basic items will comfortably support you while you are maintaining the correct physical position.

When you lie in bed for a while, in one position, your hips and legs will begin to feel very sensitive to the constant pressure against the mattress. The areas of your skin pressing against the mattress run the risk of "skin breakdown," or pressure sores. One of your first purchases will be a special pad to lay on top of your mattress and bedsheets. There are several kinds of pressure-relieving mattress overlays:

- fake fleece (washable, soft, will make you feel warm)
- foam (egg-crate mattress, spongeable, flexible for tilting)
- static air (must be checked every eight hours, creates perspiration problems from plastic surface)
- alternating air (electromechanic, needs assembly)

Mattress overlays are sold by medical supply stores and some department stores. Both have delivery service. A mattress overlay is a one-time purchase; other items may be rented from a medical supply store. Save this sales receipt and others to file medical claims or to verify medical expenses on your tax return.

Elevating Your Hips

If you need to elevate your hips above your shoulders (Trendelenburg position), you need to tilt the surface you are lying on. If you are currently using a water bed, you need to switch to a box-spring mattress. There are two ways to tilt your box-spring mattress:

1. Raise the foot end of the bed frame. That means making the two legs at the foot end taller than the two legs at the headboard. Your physician or nurse will tell you how many inches to raise the legs in order to create the right "tilt." Have a family member or friend place narrow-width solid cinder blocks or large patio flagstones, under each leg (see figures 1 and 3), making sure that the height of the blocks is the same for each leg! Don't use bricks or books. Bricks are small and can shift under the bed legs when you get in or out of bed. Books can slip away from the bed leg, creating a nasty accident.

2. A foam wedge may be a good alternative if you have a platform bed that can't be raised from the foot end. The wedge should be of the densest weight, cut to order. Your doctor or nurse

will tell you the correct measurement for the angle of the wedge. The width of the wedge should be at least half the width of the bed. This will allow you to move a bit, without changing the angle of your hips. Measure your height from your chest to your outstretched toes. The length of the wedge should be at least six inches longer than your chest-to-toes. If your wedge is too short, you'll be lying on an angle with your feet dangling in the air!

Lying on Your Side

If you have to lie on one side, you need an object to support your back. Four rolled blankets, taped securely, will be heavy enough to support you without compressing. The rolled-blanket prop has the advantage of being able to mold itself to a tilt of your bed.

An alternative object that is sturdy, rests flat on top of your mattress, and is long enough for you to rest your head, back, and buttocks is a foam bolster. A foam store can cut a bolster to fit your needs. Be sure to order the densest-weight foam for your bolster so that it will not bend or compress. See figure 2.

The height and length of the bolster is tailored to you. The height should be about two-thirds the width of your shoulders. The length is based on whether you need to lie on a tilt. If you are "tilting," the length should be equal to the top of your shoulders or your head to your hips. If you are "flat," you can make the length longer. Wrap the foam bolster in a sheet so that the inevitable spills are caught. A foam bolster can be reused after pregnancy bedrest.

I knew that when I became pregnant, I would have to lie on my side. So I ordered a foam bolster, cut to the width of my bed, sturdy enough to support me. It was so long, I needed to strap it to my car top to get it home. Amazingly, it is still a part of my bedroom eight years afterward. It rests against my headboard and I lean against it when I need to put my feet up. My daughter used it to pull herself up to stand the first time. Now the bolster supports a crowd of her Barbie dolls.

Two More Tips

Sometimes your skin becomes sensitive to the covers on top of your body. If the covers and clothes annoy you, a local appliance store can solve your problem for free. Ask for a very large packing box. Have someone cut out one long side and both ends so that the box now forms a tunnel for your legs. A hole cut in the top of the tunnel lets fresh air circulate. Now slip the box over your legs, covering your irritated parts. Place a bedsheet over the box and you can rest modestly without the irritation of clothes and sheets rubbing against your body.

Four extra pillows can increase your comfort as your pregnancy progresses beyond 20 weeks. A pillow placed between your knees takes some pressure off your hips. A small pillow placed underneath your stomach takes pressure off your back and abdominal muscles. You may need two pillows under your head to achieve a comfortable angle for reading and eating.

Sleeping Arrangements

Now that you and your bed are adjusted to maintain a specific position, your sleeping partner may have difficulty sleeping next to you. When the bed is tilted, some men have reversed positions so that their heads are higher than their feet. The foam bolster makes "three" in bed at night, and there may not be enough room for the man.

Many men are just too uncomfortable to sleep well in this situation. If you have enough space in your bedroom, consider renting a bed for your bedrest weeks. A rollaway twin cot could be used in your bedroom for your husband. You may not have enough room to open a convertible couch in your bedroom, but even a couch could serve temporarily for sleeping for you and as a sitting spot for your family and visitors.

I needed to sleep on my side, so I moved to the living-room couch at night, using its back to support my back. Once I lay down, I was "locked into" the correct bedrest position.

Actually, this separate sleeping arrangement wasn't too bad. I was closer to the bathroom for my several nightly trips. I missed my husband, but we both realized this was temporary.

Hospital Beds

Sometimes, even all the appropriate mattress overlays, bolsters, and pillows are not sturdy enough to support you in the correct position. If you are truly too uncomfortable with these arrangements, discuss with your doctor or nurse the possibility of prescribing the rental of a hospital bed. Hospital beds have mechanized frames that can adjust to almost any position by pressing buttons located within your arm's reach. The bed can also be raised or lowered, which makes getting into and out of the bed easier. The change in height can accommodate side tables for eating, too. Be sure to sleep with the bed completely flat. When you raise the head of the bed, make sure your buttocks are positioned exactly at the bend of the bed. Improperly positioning your body and sleeping with your head up can cause the terrible "hospital-bed backache."

Cost is a factor in the rental of a hospital bed. Be sure to resolve all costs and reimbursements for this rental with your insurance carrier before you sign a rental agreement. Your insurance carrier may want you to rent from a specific company or require certain conditions for the reimbursement of the cost of a hospital bed rental.

All Set? Not Quite

You still need to set up your second most important piece of equipment: your telephone. This is your contact with the outside world. Even before you started your bedrest, you were using the telephone at your doctor's office to make immediate arrangements.

The telephone with a special fifty-foot cord extension was my lifeline, my umbilical cord. I wanted to keep my phone with me everywhere I rested and walked. I needed to feel I could maintain contact with the world and be able to make calls at any time. I walked to the bathroom with my telephone cord. Then, I dragged my telephone to the couch. I felt better having my phone with me. I never did receive a call in the bathroom!

You need to have your telephone within your arm's reach. In the next chapter, you will read about types of tables to use at your bedside. Since your telephone will be used every day for practically every outside contact you make, you might consider the following accessories to make talking more comfortable:

• handset support device—a plastic piece that rests on your shoulder and positions the handset against your ear.
• headset—in place of the handset you hold, a lightweight earphone and voice piece that you wear on your head; used by customer-service companies.
• speakerphone—press a button on your telephone and you can talk without using the handset; will also enable your family to talk at the same time.
• extension cords—both for the handset and the telephone.
• telephone answering machine—you no longer have to pick up the phone every time it rings! You will always be able to get messages from the outside world. You will also be able to change the message if needed, especially if you need to leave suddenly.
• call-waiting service—enabling you to respond to more than one call at a time.
• cordless telephone—more expensive but handy.

6

*

Setting Up Your Room

When you are lying on your bed, flat or with your hips elevated, you see your bedroom from a different perspective. First, you realize that you are facing the bedside: it's difficult and uncomfortable to twist your head to look down to the foot end of your bed. Second, you realize that you are most comfortable looking at objects that are level with your eyes: about three feet above the floor.

Making the most of your bedsides is important for your comfort. Before the bed legs are raised, consider moving the bed so that one side faces a window. The bed might be placed on an angle in the room to take advantage of light during the day. Remember, you designed your room for bedtime; now it has to be redesigned to help you throughout the day. Being able to look out of a window and feel sunlight on your face will make you feel good and keep track of the rhythms of morning, afternoon, and evening. Figure 1 illustrates these points.

Reaching From Your Bedside

Once your bed is in the right place and your basic equipment for
your lying-down position is set up, you need to figure out how far
you can reach without stretching yourself out of position. Lying
down in the center of your bed does not enable you to reach beyond
the edge. Try to position yourself near one side of the bed so that
your arm's reach extends comfortably beyond the edge of the
mattress.

Now that you're correctly positioned, you need a flat surface
about the same height as your mattress. Your basic table belongs
within comfortable arm's reach of your bedside. This table should
have wheels so that it can be moved easily. Roller casters can be
installed on your nightstand. However, you may want to keep your
nightstand at the headboard and use other types of wheeled tables
within your arm's reach:

- television cart on wheels
- tea cart with wheels and shelves
- utility baskets, usually three tiers, and wheels
- end table on casters

Equip your rolling table with:

- telephone (see Chapter 5, "Basic Equipment")
- telephone address book
- telephone directory, on lower shelf
- radio
- Thermos, filled with a cool drink
- second Thermos, filled with hot water
- lidded cup for drinking, with hole in top for a straw (Plastic
  commuter cups have lids and straw holes. A plastic ice cream
  container or yogurt container can be washed, and a hole punched
  into the lid for your drinking.)
- package of plastic flexi-straws
- tea bags, sugar packets, jar of coffee, spoons
- picnic cooler, placed on floor or bottom shelf

- tissues
- moisturizing lotion for face and hands
- nail files, manicure items, nail clippers
- hairbrush, comb, barrettes
- mirror, preferably one on a base that can be tilted
- cleansing wipes (pop-up containers are best)
- large monthly desk calendar
- pencils, pads
- a gadget to signal your family in other parts of the home (for example, a loud ringing bell, cowbell, electric bell, or buzzer can easily be made with items from the hardware store. Or use walkie-talkies—the toys work well—or two-way talking units that plug into outlets).

Not all of these items need to be on the cart or table. You can use a set of shoe pockets to store the smaller stuff. Slide the top row of the shoe pockets underneath the mattress. Then the lower rows will hang over the side of your bed, handy for the pens, nail files, and other small things. The shoe pockets could also be fastened to the side of the cart or table.

You can extend the reach of your arm with a mechanical gripper. A gripper is a pole with tweezerlike tongs at one end and a trigger handle. When you squeeze the trigger, the tongs close around objects. Many people use grippers to reach cans on the top shelves of their kitchens. You can use a gripper to reach for items that have fallen down or to move your wheeled table.

You need two flat surfaces: one for writing or resting books, and another for holding your meals. These two flat surfaces need to be positioned right next to you when you are lying down. Both can be made quickly and cheaply.

Make your own lap desk by fastening a large clipboard or cookie sheet to a pillow. Use masking tape to strap the flat surface, or use sticky-backed Velcro pads so that the pillow can be removed easily. This lap desk molds itself to your body and can tilt in any direction. A chained pen is a nice finishing touch.

Turn your lap desk into a magnetic board. Purchase a sticky-backed activity sheet, the kind that organized people use on their refrigerator doors, and use the refrigerator magnets to secure your paperwork.

Make an eating tray that is practically spillproof by fastening a flat-bottomed roaster pan to a pillow. The sides of the roaster pan are about two inches high, easily able to hold in sloshed food and liquids. With this system, you could even risk eating soup! Sticky-backed Velcro pads can hold your pan to the pillow. Put Velcro pads on the bottom of the pan and the corresponding pads underneath your dishes. Even if the pan moves, the dishes will remain in place.

It's not really necessary, but if you have the funds, you might consider renting or purchasing an over-the-bed table. These tables are C-shaped; the bottom side is wheeled and the top of the C is a table. The C shape enables the table to slide under and over traditional four-legged beds. The problem with this table is that it is designed to be used sitting up in bed. In order for this table to be useful for you, its height should be lowered to about two inches above your mattress height. That way, you can continue to eat while maintaining your lying-down position.

A breakfast tray with legs presents the same problems as the over-the-bed table. It is also designed to be used while sitting up in bed. Lying on your side, you'll need to reach up to the height of a legged breakfast tray. If you are lying on a tilt, that legged monster is going to slide down to your chin!

For more specifics about mealtimes, see Chapter 16, "Managing Your Household."

If you have a small cassette player, keep it in arm's reach. You can easily keep music or book cassettes in a shoe pocket. After your telephone, the most important item in your room is your television set. It's going to be your window to the world. You need to be able to turn the channels and adjust the volume easily, so the television set needs to have a remote control device or be within your arm's reach. Bringing the family television set into your room also brings the family members into your room at all times. It sounds nice, but in the long run, it disrupts your own schedule.

If you can manage the expense, purchase or rent a small television set and cart. Many rental companies will include delivery and installation in their charges. This single piece of equipment will get you through many difficult days, but it is not considered a reimbursable medical expense.

A video cassette recorder (VCR) enables you to watch whatever you like, whenever you want. It is also possible to purchase or rent a video cassette player, a machine that plays but does not record. These players are much less expensive than the VCRs. If you purchase or rent, be sure to get a remote control device, preferably cordless, so you can operate the machine while in bed.

Once all your arm's-reach items are in place, you may discover you have too many electrical cords running near your bed. The television set, radio, lamps, and home monitoring equipment can overload the outlet nearest to your bed. A power strip, available in hardware stores, enables you to plug many two- and three-pronged (grounded) plugs into one flat outlet, which rests on the floor. Or, good-quality electrical extension cords can make use of an outlet in another part of your bedroom. Use painters' masking tape to secure the extension cords to the walls and duct tape when taping wires to the floor. Taping the wires eliminates a potential nasty trip-and-fall by you or your family.

Bedside Decorating

Your bedroom lighting may need to be adjusted to your daytime activities. You need a good reading light near your bed. A lamp can remain on your night table or you can install a wall-mounted swing-arm lamp near your headboard. Freestanding pole lamps can also be placed next to your head. Whatever lamp you use, it should have a light bulb bright enough for reading.

We tried a gadget that enables you to clap your hands to turn on and off electrical devices. Well, we lay on our sides, clapping like crazy. We looked like seals and our claps weren't strong enough to activate the device consistently. Maybe you will have better luck.

As we mentioned at the beginning of this chapter, when you are lying down, you are most comfortable looking at bedside objects that are about the same height as your head on a pillow—about three feet. Pictures or posters should be hung at a level you can see easily. It's nice to be able to look at landscapes. Travel agencies and foreign consulates will often mail free posters. Try to keep a rotating exhibit for yourself, changing the pictures every week or matching the pictures to the seasons.

If your wooden floors are slippery, a few well-placed rubber-bottomed bathroom mats will make your trips to the bathroom safer.

Your room will be completely redesigned when you have brought in a chair or two for your family and visitors. A comfortable armchair will be used by different members of your family for reading, eating (with snack tables), or just watching a program with you. One or two armchairs from your living room should be placed against the wall you face most often. If you have a couch that is small enough to fit in your room, you can have several visitors or room for a family member to stretch out and sleep.

How Can I Set Up This Bedroom Quickly?

Your bedrest room will take shape slowly. It may be seven to ten days until you are surrounded by all the furniture and items described in this chapter. Most difficult for you will be the desire to set up things yourself. You have to learn to be patient with your family and friends who will be doing all the legwork purchasing, delivering, and setting up your room.

The first days of your bedrest will be a "make-do" situation, using pillows and rolled covers to support your back and raise your hips. Medical supply stores will deliver your mattress overlay. Your phoned request to a foam store will be filled as quickly as possible if you explain your medical situation. Try to group what you need by the store that stocks it. For example, a family member or friend can shop in a hardware store for extension cords, cinder blocks, a flat electrical outlet, roller casters, magnetic tape, magnet boards, electrical tape, a gripper, and a roaster pan.

Make a diagram of your room the way you would like it, and let your family and friends follow your drawing, not your shouted directions. In fact, if your family has assembled to work on your room, move yourself to another area of your home, lie down, and take a nap!

By the end of the first week, and during the second week, you will begin to use your bedside items effectively and develop a daily schedule. During your second week you will feel comfortable reaching, eating, and sleeping. But boredom is always present, and you may begin to wonder if you could use other areas of your home for your lying-down time.

We, the authors, have never been able to agree about whether you should have more than one resting place, or nesting area, in your home. One of us always lists all the reasons to remain in the bedroom: you have to duplicate your basic equipment, movement will encourage movement, you may begin to move around from nesting area to nesting area. The other author then lists all the good reasons to create a second nest: relief from the boredom of the bedroom, more contact with the family, and the duplication of basic equipment is not difficult.

The fact that we always disagree should be your cue that the decision to create a second nesting area in your home is specific to your medical complication and family situation. We recommend that you talk to your doctor, nurse, or occupational therapist about the pros and cons of nesting areas for you.

We do agree about one issue: if you have other children, caring for them may require setting up more than one permanent resting area. The next chapter focuses on setting up rooms when you have children.

7

*

Setting Up Your
Room for Children

Your bedrest room should be accessible to your child or children, but remain their mother's room. They should feel comfortable coming into your room, have a variety of activities they can do with you, but not be able to do activities that will make you become nervous or worried.

It is extremely important to childproof your bedrest room. All electrical wires and the extension cords for your equipment should be taped to the floor edge against the walls, away from their feet and hands. Unused outlets should have childproof caps. Cover the stone blocks under the bed legs with rolled towels to prevent banged toes when your child runs around the bed. Place furniture in front of your window so that a young child will be unable to climb onto the windowsill.

When You and Your Children Are Alone
Together

The ideal situation is to have someone in your home throughout the day, who can be your "arms and legs." A family member or a paid individual can feed your children, play with them, and even take them to a playground. Many bedresters cannot afford the cost of a full-time paid caregiver or do not have relatives who are available every day, during the day, for their children. We do recommend that you try to have a second adult in your home with you and your children as often as you can manage.

When you must be the only adult at home with your children, your first concern is their safety. You keep them safe when you keep them in the same room with you. This room can be your regular bedrest room with some modifications, or you can create a second bedrest nest in the children's play area. Either room should have childproof gates at the doors to prevent your young children from leaving.

You also need to lie on a flat surface that is closer to the floor than your bed. If you are lying down about twelve inches above the floor, you can rest your young child on the floor to change a diaper. You are also at a perfect height to play with your young child. A second mattress placed on the floor will work well. A camp cot will also lower your resting position to above the floor and can be folded away when not in use. A three-section foam chair that unfolds into a bed can also be used. You might also consider using an inflatable beach raft, although the plastic surface reflects your body heat and you may perspire after lying on it for long periods of time. Some bedresters have used the couch in the living room or den as their resting place, too.

After your children spend several hours in one room, they will want to go out and play. You may try to reschedule their days so that they have a quiet time during the day with you and then can have an active evening. A trip to the supermarket with a family member can be fun in the evening. Older children will enjoy bowling, swimming, ice-skating, or just walking in a park with their father or one of your friends. Your school-age children can do their homework in the afternoon in your room or nearby and then have their active playtime in the evening.

Eating Together

Your young child's food should be prepared by another family member or caregiver. If you must feed your child alone, your child's lunch and yours should be packed in a picnic cooler, placed where you can reach it easily.

If you wish to use your sitting and standing privileges to feed your child, you can continue to use a standard high chair for feeding. The height of a high chair and the arm and body movements needed to feed a child require you to sit, move, and reach in different directions. This is active work.

Positioning your child in a chair requires reaching down and picking up your child. Talk to your doctor about this special lifting and be sure to say how much your child weighs. You need to lift your child out of playpens, too. It is important to discuss with your nurse and doctor the specifics of what you can and can't do in caring for your child.

An alternative to the high chair is the close-to-the-ground feeding table. This is a table about thirty inches high that has roller-caster legs. The child's seat is in the middle of the table. The seat back may fold over to create a large play table, too. When your child is sitting at this lower height, you can more easily reach across and down to him. But even helping your child eat at a feeding table is an active activity for you.

A high-chair safety harness or an over-the-chair child fabric seat can be used to secure your young child to a child's seat or a full-sized chair. A child's play table and chair can then become a feeding table.

An ironing board can be shared by you and your young child. The height of the board is adjusted so that it rests on top of your mattress. The length of the ironing board is slipped over the bedside, creating one long supported flat surface. Your young child, secured to a full-size chair, faces you. Food or play objects are spread along this long flat surface. Cover the board with a washable plastic cloth. See figure 2.

Your older child can eat at a card table or folding snack table at your bedside. When you eat with your older child, push away the bedside tables so that your child is sitting next to you. Your child will eat, seeing Mommy using her hands, laughing, and asking questions about school. When your child sits at the end of your bed, it's difficult to turn your head to see him. From the foot end of the bed, your child will see you lying in bed, a sick parent. Keep your child close to minimize this anxiety-producing image of you. See figure 4, on p. 45.

Playtime

Watching television together counts as playtime. When you both watch an educational program such as "Sesame Street," or any commercial programs your young child enjoys, you are doing something together. You can count together, recite the alphabet, or you can ask your child about the characters in the television program. One of the advantages of watching these children's programs is that they are funny, and laughing together is good for both of you.

Your young child and you can play together at the feeding table or share the ironing board. Toys that are attached to strings tied to the chair eliminate reaching down for your toddler's version of catch.

If your child plays in a playpen, you need to be able to watch her play at all times as well as reach over the edge. You might think about keeping one edge of a mesh playpen collapsed down, but don't do it. Children can get caught in the folded mesh—a nasty accident. An inexpensive closet mirror can be an interesting alternative. Place it on a wall next to the playpen, tilted so that it reflects the bottom of the playpen. Then you can look at the mirror and see your child play. Even with this help, you should expect that having your child play next to you is active work for you.

In the previous chapter, we described the mechanical gripper that enables you to extend your reach. It's a valuable tool for reaching bottles, spoons, and toys that are on the floor or in the playpen.

- Store playtime objects in an inexpensive cardboard storage chest.
- A set of shoe pockets hung on a wall can be used by an older child to store crayons, scissors, and books.

- Tape the outline of a refrigerator to one wall of your room to display your child's artwork.
- A nice addition to your room is a fish tank. It is interesting for you and your children to observe and it is a nice way to teach your children how to take care of a pet. Even a small child can tap some fish flakes into the tank. Be sure that the electrical filter equipment is safely out of your child's reach.

Reading Together

A table or a shelf in your room can be used for your child's books. Reading to your child requires no special equipment other than a good reading lamp and room enough on your bed for your child to snuggle up.

Naptime

You may try to arrange for your child to be cared for outside of your home or in your home for part of the day. Then, the part of the day you are alone together will hopefully be your child's naptime. If your child is most comfortable sleeping in his own bed, "gate" the doorway, and install a walkie-talkie or listening device so that you can hear him wake up. You might want to arrange your day so that you nap when your child is away and are fully refreshed and awake when your child is napping.

If your child will be napping in your bedroom, be sure your room is gated. You can share a mattress on the floor, or remain on your bed while your child sleeps on a camp cot. It's also a good idea to have a midday snack within arm's reach of your napping area. Juice boxes and cookies can be placed in your child's room or next to your bed.

Schoolwork

Your young school-age child can complete homework assignments at your bedside. The card table or snack table next to you will work well. Your child can borrow your lap desk or make a second one. A shoe pocket tacked to the arm of a chair can hold extra school supplies.

Your older child may want to work in another room, her bedroom or the kitchen. If your child comes home from school and spends time in another area of the home, buying walkie-talkies for long-distance conversations is necessary. Your child can then carry her device to any part of the home.

An older child has outgrown the need for "refrigerator art" and now has a complicated weekly schedule of school and outside activities. Get a very large weekly planner to hang on the wall near your bedside. Your older child can write in the activities and you can work on arranging car pools, calling teachers, and helping him get ready for a school test. Or your older child can write her activities on seven large paper sheets, taped to the side wall so you can read each "day sheet" while lying in bed. When your older child sees this visible proof that her activities have an important place in your life and that you are doing your best to participate and to help her, your high-risk pregnancy will become less frightening and more a temporarily difficult situation that her mother is handling.

How Your Room Looks to Your Child

Your bedroom has always been a special grown-up place for your children. The curtains, bedspread, lamps all mean "parents" to them. Children like to play in a parent's room, fingering the perfume bottles and brushes, making grown-up faces in the mirror.

Now all of that has changed. In redesigning your room for bedrest, you moved or put away many personal things. Your room looks strange and unfamiliar. During your first days of bedrest, your young child may hesitate at the doorway, not wanting to enter a room filled with carts, equipment, and a bed tilted on an angle.

If every wall is covered with drawings and the floor is scattered with toys, the room will still look unfamiliar, not like a parent's room. Your bedrest room should have the pictures and decorations that reflect your grown-up taste and style. The "artwork" and

schoolwork should have one place in the room, and the play supplies should be put away when not in use. Just as you are gradually
getting used to this situation, your child needs some time to adjust
to Mother's bedrest room. During the first few days, just sitting in
an armchair near you, watching a television program, will help
accustom your child to being in the room. He will feel confused if
his table and chairs are quickly moved from his room to yours. It's
better to wait a few days and make this change when it makes sense
to him. As you get used to your room and become more skilled in
reaching for items near you, your child will get used to these
changes, too. In fact, it's not unusual for a child to make a few
adjustments in your room that make you more comfortable!

> My six-year-old liked sitting on his school chair while we
> watched "He Man." One day he moved his chair against the
> bed so that he and I could face the television set while I lay
> on my side. Then he said, "Mom, hold onto my chair when
> you get out of bed." He was right; when he sat on the chair, I
> could put my hand on the chair back to help steady myself
> when I stood up. I was so proud of him.

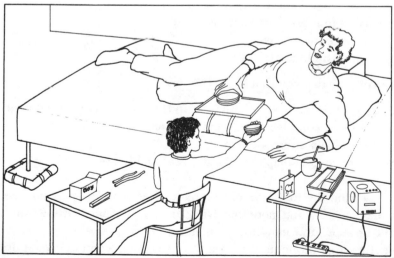

Fig. 4

8

*

Planning Your Days

Every day of your therapeutic pregnancy bedrest should begin with:

1. an early awakening (by 7:30 A.M.)
2. a complete breakfast (not just coffee)
3. a change into daywear
4. washup and hairstyling

During the day you should:

5. take a brief shower or bath (within the limits set by your doctor)
6. eat three complete meals and two snacks
7. take a brief afternoon nap
8. get ready for sleep at night at a reasonable hour.

During the first days of pregnancy bedrest, you may not feel like doing anything more than lying on your bed and drifting in and out of naps. You may put off making plans until after your next doctor's appointment, after you have the room completely set up, or after you have gotten used to bedrest.

It is easy, all too easy, just to lie in bed and let yourself go. No matter what else you are able to do during these first few days, force yourself to complete these eight tasks. They will make you feel awake, refreshed, and actually less restless when you are lying down.

Push yourself to keep to a schedule. If your bedrest day has an order to it, you will feel better physically and emotionally.

Break up your day into smaller periods: times for each meal, for snacks, television programs, reading, naps, telephone calling. A day that has a schedule seems to pass more quickly than a day you plan as you go along.

A day that has a schedule, filled with set times for set activities, fights off the boredom that can lead to depression. Developing a plan for the day will enable you to learn how to balance your lying-down time with the time you are allowed for sitting up and for walking to the bathroom.

Force yourself to begin to write down all your daily activities on a calendar. If you are a list maker, develop a daily list of things to do and check them off, just as you do when you are active.

Here's a list of what belongs on a daily bedrest schedule:

- Meals. You may be allowed to sit up or eat with the family. Make sure your time for eating is within the limits set by your doctor. Your family should follow this schedule to help you. Stick to a specific time for your snacks.
- Bathroom privileges. If you are allowed a brief daily shower, or three showers each week, schedule these times so that you are not alone in the home while you are standing up and so that your looked-forward-to shower does not clash with your teenager's preparation for a date.
- Afternoon nap. You do need a rest time, even when you are lying down. An hour's break in the day, perhaps early in the afternoon, will quiet your mind and prepare you for an evening of activities with your family. The nap can also get you through the afternoon blahs—a common low point in the bedrester day.
- Telephone calls. Try to make phone calls, not receive them. You will need to do a lot of telephone business: setting up appoint-

ments, talking to your doctor and nurse, shopping by phone, talking to your work supervisor or your child's teacher. Personal phone calls to friends and relatives should also be planned. Make sure your friends and family know when you are "talking" and what times you are napping.

- Medical tests. You may be required to do some simple observations of how you feel and of fetal movements during each day. Some women are required to use home monitoring equipment each day and transmit that information to a medical office. This time may be preset by your doctor or your nurse. Be sure to discuss with your nurse what activities you should avoid before a medical test.
- Television and radio time. Become an active watcher; don't just lie there and let the television blare. Read the channel listings and write down the times of programs you want to watch. Or record a television program and watch it at a time that is best for you and your family. One woman recorded a full week of her favorite soap opera and watched with her friend on Saturday morning instead of cartoons!
- Your children's hour. Plan a time each day for homework, play, even for your children's favorite evening show.
- Activity time. Whether it's reading a book, doing a craft, writing a letter, or listening to music, you need time each day to do *something* for yourself. See Chapter 17, "Expanding Your Horizons."

It can also be helpful to solve your daily problems and make plans by thinking of the seven C's of pregnancy bedrest. They are listed below along with the chapter in which each subject is discussed.

Clothes	Chapter 10
Chores	Chapter 16
Child care	Chapters 7 and 25
Contacts	Chapters 18 and 26
Costs	Chapters 14 and 15
Couples	Chapters 22, 23, 24
Crafts	Chapter 17

Force yourself to make plans beyond each day—to plan for an entire week or a full month ahead. A monthly planner, desk size, is a terrific help to manage your bedrest time. What belongs on your monthly planner?

- Your doctor's appointments. Use your desk calendar to write the dates and times for your next three appointments. Now, when you look at your calendar, your bedrest time is divided into the times between appointments.
- Entertainment. With your doctor's permission, you may be allowed to have visitors. Force yourself to plan two weeks ahead.
- Count off the time until your due date. Many bedresters marked their desk calendars with the weeks until their due dates. Some counted forward and some counted backward; for example, a woman on bedrest for three weeks, at week 28 of her pregnancy, might say:

   "I've finished 3 weeks on bedrest, I'm at 28 weeks in this pregnancy, 9 weeks until the first week of full term at 37 weeks." Or,

   "When I started bedrest at 25 weeks, my doctor told me I needed 12 weeks lying on a tilt to reach 37 weeks, full term. Well, I finished 12, 11, 10, and now I'm down to week 9."
- Achievement days. Every day that you maintain yourself on bedrest is a victory for you and for your baby. A full week completed deserves some congratulations. These bedresters developed their own rewards:

   "I sliced a black forest cake into ten sections, one for each week I needed to be on bedrest. The slices were wrapped and frozen; on Saturday night, a slice was defrosted and was my special dessert."

   "I had a friend paste a wall full of those yellow sticky-backed pads—one for each day I had to be on bedrest. Every morning I ripped off one on the way to the bathroom. It was silly, but when I was able to eliminate an entire row, I felt great!"

How Your Family Feels about Your
Schedule

Before you started bedrest, you and your family raced through each day and each week, juggling work, car pools, birthday parties, and baby-sitters. Suddenly, your family has to continue their daily work and play without your help. And they have to do many things that you used to do, like grocery shopping, driving kids to a soccer game, or buying a birthday gift. You can still participate in many family activities by being the person who does the telephone work. You can become the parent scheduler for car pools and baby-sitting co-ops. A craft project can become a very special birthday gift to give. You can write the shopping lists, trade coupons, and locate the lowest prices for your family shopping trips.

Since you are lying in one place, at home, your family members now see you as someone who can answer their questions at any time of the day, who can adapt herself to any changes because all she has to do is continue to lie in bed.

But you have your own schedule, too. For all the reasons you read above, you need to develop and stick to a routine each day. Your family has to support your effort to manage your bedrest by following your meal times, nap times, and medical test times.

During the first days of your bedrest, when everyone is rearranging their routines and schedules, you should be working on your bedrest schedule, too. A family that creates a new schedule together is a family that maintains that new schedule better.

9

※

Bathroom Privileges

In the previous chaptor, you read about the eight basic tasks to do each day. This short chapter is about task 4, washup and hairstyling, and task 5, taking a brief shower or bath.

Many personal grooming tasks can be done while you are in bed. You can file your nails, pluck your eyebrows, and style your hair. You can also apply moisturizing lotions to your body.

Your skin will quickly feel the effects of being indoors and lying down. It may become dry and sensitive. Rough spots may develop on parts of your body that press against the bed. Keep your skin elastic and soft by applying lotions several times each day. You will feel much more comfortable if you are given a once-a-day application of lotion on your back and legs. You may need to switch from using a soap to a gentle cleanser.

You won't be getting much sunlight on your body for a while, so your skin will be its palest shade. But look at it this way, you'll be missing a few weeks of the sun's rays that promote wrinkles. You will also be more sensitive to these rays when you are back on your feet again. If you finish your pregnancy in the warmer months, remember to use a good sun-block lotion when you are outside.

Some pleasant self-care can be started while in bed and finished in your bathroom. You can apply a facial mask while in bed and then peel or wash it off when you go to the bathroom.

Keep some daywear and nightgowns hanging in your bathroom. An over-the-door hook will keep changes of clothes neatly hung. As soon as you finish your washup or shower, your clothes will be in arm's reach.

Since bathrooms are the primary place for slipping accidents in a home, make sure you have a rubber mat in your tub or shower stall and that the bathroom floor is covered with nonskid materials. Do you have something to hold onto when you get in and out of the tub? A bathroom handgrip can be installed on the wall to make climbing out of the tub safer.

When you stand up after using the toilet, remember the eight steps you follow when getting out of bed. Be sure to use a sturdy object, like the sink top, to help steady you when you push yourself to a standing position.

How often you are allowed to take baths or showers is decided by your doctor based on your medical condition. For example, you might be allowed a ten-minute shower every other day. You may be allowed to take tub baths. When you do shower or bathe, it is a good idea to have a family member close by to help you get in and out of the tub.

It is important to note here that if you are experiencing any light-headedness or dizziness when you change positions, you may also find that *very hot* showers make you feel faint.

Now to the most important issue: hair care!

Shampooing your hair in the shower requires you to stand up for a longer time than just washing. Consider purchasing a special chair made for placement in a tub or shower stall. These chairs, sold in medical supply stores, look just like ordinary chairs, except they are extremely sturdy and meet the specifications of insurance carriers. Keep the receipt for your medical insurance and income tax files. Sitting while you shampoo may seem a little silly at first, but you will be much more comfortable.

If your shower privileges do not extend to washing your hair, you have two alternatives. Your first is to use a "dry shampoo." This is actually a lotion made of the same ingredients as strong alcohol-based astringents used to tighten facial pores. The lotion is applied to your scalp with cotton balls and rinsed out by wringing your hair in a wet towel. Before you attempt to use a dry shampoo, let your doctor or nurse read the label of the product to make sure you can safely apply it to your hair and your scalp.

Your second alternative is to purchase a special shampoo tray. One commercial brand is called Shampeeze. This tray rests on your shoulders and extends outward so that all water can be directed to a large bucket. To wash your hair, you lie on your back, rest your shoulders on the tray, and have your helper place a large bucket underneath your head. Your helper then uses a small bucket of fresh water to wet your hair and rinse the soap down the tray into the receiving bucket. This special tray can be purchased from a beauty supply store.

In addition to getting dirty, your hair will continue to grow throughout your bedrest pregnancy. At the same time, your face will change a bit as you progress in your pregnancy. A haircut, even just a trim, will boost your spirits.

Often, nurses can provide referrals to hairstylists who work in hospitals and are experienced in giving haircuts to people who are lying in bed. Of course, you may wish to keep your current hairstylist and that person may be happy to help you by coming to your home. But make sure that stylist understands your current limitations.

Once you do arrange for an appointment, have the stylist phone you when he or she is about to travel to your home—even if you have a set time for an appointment. You know how hectic a hair salon can be. Home haircuts are more expensive than salon service, so be sure to understand exactly what you will be charged and the best method of payment.

10

*

Your Wardrobe

Every book about pregnancy contains a chapter about the special clothing a pregnant woman needs. You need the same kinds of underwear and much the same kind of clothes. We will be referring to clothes here as daywear, nightwear, and for office visits. We are also going to describe how to buy clothes and how to get your clothes altered.

This chapter may not make much sense to you right now. If you've just gotten started on bedrest, you are probably wearing your nightgown as you are reading this book. What are they talking about? you're wondering. I'll spend this pregnancy in bed. Why do I need to wear clothes?

But think about the last time you wore your nightgown during the day. You were sick with a sore throat or flu, too ill to go out to work. So, you got up, put on your bathrobe, called your office, then walked back into your bedroom, took off your robe, and went back to sleep. Only when you started to feel better, or were trying to make yourself feel better, did you change out of your nightgown into a sweatshirt and pants. And when your family saw you in your sweats, they probably said, "Hey, you must be feeling better!"

Wearing your nightgown during the day is going to make you

look like a sick person to your family and to yourself. You are not sick; you are pregnant with a medical condition that requires lying down for periods of time. So keep your nightgowns for the night-time and begin each day by changing into pregnancy day clothes that are comfortable for lying down.

If you have bathroom privileges, try to have your day outfit hanging in the bathroom so that you can combine your standing time and morning washing with changing into fresh clothes. You may want to have breakfast in bed and then wash so that you are refreshed and ready when you return to the bed. During that time, a family member can air out the room, open a window, even remake the bed.

DAYWEAR

- 4 cotton/acrylic drawstring sweatpants. These can be maternity sweat pants or regular, just size extra-large. If the elastic leg bottoms begin to irritate your ankles, just open a seam and remove the elastic ring.
- 5–6 T-shirts. You can wear maternity tops or use men's T-shirts, size extra-large. If this size is still tight, cut side vents. One woman used fabric marker pens to decorate several men's under-shirts.
- 5–6 pairs of underpants. You will need maternity underpants, which are specifically designed to your changing size. Or, during the later weeks, low-slung bikini underpants can fit comfortably below your belly.
- 2–3 maternity bras.
- 1 pair of shoes to wear for bathroom privileges. This pair can be slippers or your most comfortable slip-on shoes.

NIGHTWEAR

- 6–7 nightgowns. Sleeveless gowns will be looser around your arms and chest. Large-size sleep shirts work well, too.
- maternity bras. You may feel better wearing a bra during the night.

• 1 lightweight wrapper robe. A large-size kimono wrapper is a good investment for homewear and to take to the hospital.

OFFICE VISITS

• 2 pregnancy outfits to buy or borrow. Since this is your only outing, select an outfit that makes you feel dressed up.
• 2–3 pairs of maternity pantyhose.
• 1 maternity slip (you already have the underpants).
• your most comfortable slip-on shoes. No, not the high-heeled pumps! Dress shoes should be low-heeled so you don't tip forward when you walk.
• a tote bag for carrying specimens, notepads, snacks.
• a cape, poncho, large wool wrap. You will be outside very briefly, traveling from your home to the doctor's office. Don't wear any outer clothes that are heavy to carry around when you are indoors. Besides, what pregnant woman is cold?

Buying Your Clothes

You can manage most of the "footwork" of shopping for your clothes. Many department store catalogues have sections for maternity clothes. And maternity stores now offer catalogue service, too. All you need to do is write down the appropriate catalogue numbers and dial the customer-service number.

Your maternity underwear size is based on your nonpregnant sizes. So write down your nonpregnant dimensions before you phone.

Perhaps you spent some time looking at maternity clothes in a local store before you were told you would be on bedrest. And now you would still like to buy one outfit you saw and liked. Phone the store and explain to the saleswoman your current situation. She can assemble that specific outfit based on your nonpregnant size, and collect other items you need. Be sure to ask for an outfit in at least two different sizes or select a second backup dress. A family member or a friend can go to the store and buy the clothes (and return what is not wanted).

Use your standing-up time to try on these clothes. Have a full-length mirror nearby. Then be sure to have the clothes you don't want returned within the refund time limit. It's that simple.

By the way, fathers make great shoppers. When a man enters a maternity department and explains why the mother of his child cannot shop herself, he will receive quick and attentive help. You may find that he picked out and brought home a few bonus clothing items he thought you would like.

Alterations

When you try on a maternity dress, have some straight pins nearby. Your clothes helper, standing nearby, can quickly pin the hem to the length you want. Maternity dresses have hems that are longer in the front than at the sides. As your stomach grows, the hem is raised so that it is even all around. So pin up a side section first and judge the length of the dress by that.

The hemming should be done by someone who has experience in this work. Maternity shops often have their own tailors or refer customers to certain tailor shops. If you purchased your dress by mail, a local maternity shop may do the alteration for a small charge or provide a good referral.

The hemming of maternity pants is easier. Match the inseam of pregnancy pants with the inseam of a pair of pants you wore before your pregnancy. After you've pinned the pregnancy pants to the same length, pull them on and slip on your pregnancy outdoor shoes. Pregnancy pants will fit a bit differently, so you may want to adjust the hem length a second time. The hemming of a pants leg is a simple job—a good opportunity to teach your child to sew. Your child can hem one leg while you hem the other.

What can you do if you are not allowed sufficient time to try on maternity outfits? This is tricky, but you can manage it. If you want a dress, try to pick out a soft sleeveless jumper. If the width of your shoulders and the width between the jumper shoulder straps is roughly the same, you've got a fit. T-shirts worn with a jumper look good. A tailor can raise the hem without a pinup by comparing one of your nonpregnancy dresses to match lengths. Pregnancy pants have the advantage in this situation.

When Your Shoes Don't Fit

A very common experience during pregnancy is discovering that your shoes are too tight. Your feet do tend to expand during a pregnancy. This slight expansion is different from the swollen ankles and puffiness that is a warning signal. Your feet expand in width, not in length. One pair of leather shoes can be chemically stretched by a shoemaker. Or, purchase the same style and length you like but go one letter size wider (from 8A to 8B, for example). A pair of sandals with leather straps will stretch a bit, too.

*

YOUR MEDICAL
MANAGEMENT
TEAM

*

11

*

Working with
Your Doctor

The management of your bedrest pregnancy requires a special kind of teamwork between you and your doctor. You will be working each day to maintain your specific lying-down position and to stay within your limits for sitting-up and standing privileges. Your doctor must use skills and experience in monitoring your medical condition. You will be referred to other health professionals for medical tests in order to gain more information about your pregnancy as it progresses.

Your role is to become an active patient, supplying your doctor and other health professionals with accurate information about yourself to help in the assessment of your medical condition. Becoming an active patient does not mean that you must read medical journals or even fully understand all the aspects of your specific medical complication. Becoming an active patient means developing the ability to be aware of how you feel and being able to communicate this to your doctor during your office visits and by telephone.

When You Are Treated by a New Doctor

Sometimes, your current doctor may recommend that your high-risk pregnancy be managed by a specialist in the field of pregnancy complications. A doctor who practices in the field of high-risk pregnancies is called a maternal-fetal medicine specialist or perinatologist. This doctor heads a team of health professionals that see patients in an outpatient clinic of a large medical center. This medical center may be the regional perinatal center for treatment of all high-risk patients in a geographical area. Changing doctors, coming at a time when you are receiving the news that your pregnancy has a serious problem, can completely overwhelm you. While you are trying to deal with all the impossible tasks of beginning pregnancy bedrest, you have to travel to a new medical office and be treated by a doctor you've never met.

Your anger at everything that is happening to you is often directed at the medical staff in this outpatient clinic. You may want to cooperate but, at the same time, feel mistrustful of the new staff people who are treating you. Your new doctor and the office staff are aware of your mixed feelings. Practically every woman patient sitting in the outpatient waiting room with you feels just the same way. Specialists in the field of high-risk-pregnancy management are very sensitive to the special needs of their patients. You will find that their awareness of your feelings and physical discomforts is usually very supportive.

Office Visits

It seems like a contradiction: first your doctor tells you that you must lie down for part or most of the day and restricts all your sitting up and standing to specified times. Then you are scheduled for more office visits!

You might think that an old-fashioned house call might be more appropriate. Some bedresters do receive house calls from trained nurses (described in the next chapter). But, your doctor must be able to examine you in an office that has a medical laboratory, examination tables, and diagnostic equipment. An examination for a high-risk pregnancy requires a fully equipped examination room and special medical equipment.

You can minimize the physical stress of going to these appointments by scheduling your visits for the same weekday at the same time. For example, if you need to see the doctor once a week, try to schedule each appointment for the same time on the same day. This steady schedule will get you into a routine for dressing, traveling, and resting afterward. You also need to develop a steady routine for the person who will be taking you to the clinic and getting you back to your home. Bedresters should make all efforts to get help in traveling to their appointments, even arranging for taxi service.

The same-day, same-time appointments also provide the best data for your doctor. Many physical changes in your medical condition are progressive; changes occur at a certain rate throughout your pregnancy. Weight gain is a good example. If you are able to be weighed on a regular basis, once a week, your doctor can accurately measure the rate at which you are gaining weight.

Try to schedule your office appointments at least four weeks in advance. This saves time for the office secretary and enables you and your family to plan ahead. Thinking four weeks forward is a way of concentrating on short-term goals. Instead of thinking about the time until your due date, concentrate on the days between each weekly appointment.

The Day Before Your Office Visit

Write down all the questions you want to ask your doctor. Review this list with your family (children included). They might remember some questions you've forgotten and they might have questions of their own.

Lenette Moses, of Intensive Caring Unlimited, prepared a wonderful checklist for women to take to their doctors. It is reprinted in Appendix 3. Remember that as your pregnancy progresses, your lying-down, sitting-up, and standing privileges will be adjusted. Review this checklist with your doctor periodically.

Your questions will do more than reassure you and your family. They are a clue as to how you are feeling. A doctor is trained to use the patient's questions to help diagnose a medical complication. So your long list of questions is an important source of information for your doctor.

Decide which of the one or two outfits you are going to wear and make sure all your inner and outer clothes are clean and ready. It is not unusual for a bedrest patient to be admitted to the hospital from the doctor's office, so have a hospital bag packed and ready, waiting by your front door in plain sight or packed in the trunk of the family car.

The Morning of Your Appointment

Pack your visit tote bag with your list of questions, pen and paper for writing down information, and something to keep you occupied if you need to wait at the office.

Dress slowly. Allow enough time so that after you are dressed, you can lie down again for a while.

Traveling to Your Appointment

If you are still allowed to drive, try to give yourself enough time to drive slowly to the doctor's office. You need a few extra minutes to reorient yourself to being outside and sitting behind the wheel.

If you have passenger privileges only, wait until your transportation is at the door with the motor running to close your front door behind you. Then carefully get into the car or taxi.

As always, seat belts are very important. Dr. David Nagey, the Director of Maternal Fetal Medicine at the University of Maryland School of Medicine, says, "Automobile accidents are a significant risk during any pregnancy, and one of every two hundred admissions to our Shock/Trauma Unit is pregnant! Bedrester or not, a pregnant woman should wear her belts properly, which turns out to be identical to the proper way for anyone to wear seat belts. The lap belt should be as low as possible and as tight as comfortably possible. In an accident the belt must protect the pelvic girdle. The shoulder harness must be worn and should be loose enough to admit a fist between the breastbone and the belt. In other words, in an accident, the woman's chest should have an inch or two to move forward before being stopped by the belt. In a car without shoulder harnesses, it is next safest to ride in the back seat, perhaps lying down with no belt. The danger is that a lap belt alone can, in an accident, cause the pregnant woman to 'jackknife' about the lap belt, compressing all her intraabdominal organs including the uterus, perhaps leading to uterine rupture or rupture of the liver, spleen or aorta. The safest, however, is to ride with both lap belt and shoulder harness worn as described above."

During Your Appointment

Waiting rooms have only chairs. If your appointment is delayed or you are feeling a little light-headed, ask to wait for your doctor in an examination room where you can lie down on the examination table until your doctor arrives.

Be aware of yourself. Your doctor will ask you how you feel and what physical changes you have experienced since the last appointment. The better you can communicate what you are experiencing, the better your doctor can evaluate your medical condition.

Every pregnant woman senses changes in her body as her baby is growing. You will be especially aware of these physical changes and fetal movements because you are lying quietly in bed. At the same time, you will be anxious and worried about every movement and twinge you feel. It is not easy, but it is important to separate what you are actually experiencing physically from your fears and fantasies.

I decided to keep a daily diary. Every day, right after my nap, I wrote two or three sentences about the day. Tuesday, it might be "feeling nauseous," or "kid is hiccuping after meals." Some days I just wrote, "Feeling lousy." After a few weeks, I noticed that some days I felt lousy and then in a few days I would feel great. So there was a pattern to how I was feeling. There was a definite pattern to the hiccups. My doctor appreciated this information and I was less nervous when I had a lousy day.

After your examination is completed, stop by the billing office and submit a medical claim form for the appointment. Don't leave the office until you feel ready to drive. If your transportation is delayed, try to lie down in a vacant room.

The Evening After Your Appointment

You will be tired. Traveling to a medical office, being examined, and waiting for reassuring news from your doctor is an exhausting experience. Many bedresters come home from their appointments and promptly take naps. Review the answers to your questions with your family. Share the good news and don't hold back on any new problems.

Warning Signals

There are standard warning signals that are symptoms of medical problems for every pregnancy. And then there are the warning signals for *your* pregnancy. Your doctor will tell you about certain changes in how you feel, physical sensations, and vaginal discharges that are warning signals of changes in your specific medical condition. Your role in the medical management of your pregnancy is to fully understand your warning signals and to know how to contact your doctor quickly.

Learn your doctor's office hours and what telephone numbers to call in the evening and during the night. If your doctor is on rotation or takes turns with other doctors to receive calls in the evening, make sure that these other doctors also understand your medical condition.

Prepare yourself for an emergency admission to the hospital. Write a quick history of this pregnancy and the medical complications you have. Include your doctor's telephone number and the medical insurance identification. Keep one copy of this history in your hospital bag and the second copy in your purse—the purse you always carry with you.

What if you are concerned or have a question and you are not experiencing a warning signal? Are you bothering your doctor if you call more than once a week?

You shouldn't hesitate to call your doctor about any concern you have. You don't know how upset you are feeling until you hear some reassuring answers to your questions. But not every question is an emergency. Work out a system with your doctor to express the degree of your concern when you call. Above all, trust your feelings when you feel the need to get in touch with your doctor.

12

*

Working with
Your Nurse

Throughout your bedrest pregnancy, you will talk to and be cared for by nurses who specialize in maternal-fetal medicine. There is a special quality of caring that these nurses provide for their patients. Most likely your nurse will be a woman, and you will need and appreciate being able to talk woman-to-woman about your high-risk pregnancy. At times you may well feel more comfortable talking to your nurse than to your doctor. That's one of the reasons that the management of a high-risk pregnancy requires the teamwork of doctors and nurses as well as other health professionals.

This teamwork of doctors and nurses is also a result of the specialized education and training that nurses have nowadays. Your nurse provides skilled, specialized care in administering medications and monitoring their effect on you. During the beginning of an office visit, your nurse will perform some initial tests, take your vital signs, and ask you how you are feeling and what physical changes you are experiencing. If you are being examined by a nurse practitioner, she may perform a complete physical assessment and propose treatments in conjunction with your doctor's medical diagnosis.

Your nurse is the health professional who will teach you the nuts and bolts of pregnancy bedrest. She will teach you how to position yourself when you are lying down. You and your nurse will review together the checklists in the Appendix of this book. Your questions about bathroom privileges, mealtimes, and the care of your other children will be directed to your nurse.

You might receive a home visit from a nurse. Your visiting nurse may examine you, perform a diagnostic test, and be in contact with your doctor. But a home visit is also a chance for you and your nurse to talk about all the daily issues of managing your bedrest. This visitor understands what you are experiencing and can provide helpful advice,

Your nurse often communicates with other staff members of the clinic, hospital, or in private practice, to provide advice about exercise, diet, and concrete medical and social services. Your nurse will help maintain your diet program, make sure you are performing physical therapy exercises correctly, and even help you to complete the forms you need to obtain state and local assistance.

Nursing really has changed greatly since your mother was pregnant with you. Most nurses still dress in white, although many now wear comfortable pants and tops rather than uniform dresses. Their shoes are still sturdy and white but now look more like your aerobic shoes. Some nurses even have their own offices. In your mother's day, a nurse's cap identified what school she had attended. Now the identification badge that a nurse wears can tell you what undergraduate and graduate degrees she holds. Here are some of the initials you may see on her badge:

R.N.	registered nurse
B.S.N.	bachelor of science in nursing
M.S.N.	masters of science in nursing
Ph.D.	doctorate in nursing
R.N.C.	registered nurse certified
C.N.M.	certified nurse midwife
R.N.P.	registered nurse practitioner

C.R.N.A.   certified registered nurse anesthetist

L.P.N.   licensed practical nurse

Nurses have different job titles and job descriptions. Here are some of the different nurses who will care for you:

Clinical Nurse: a nurse who performs direct nursing care in hospitals, clinics, outpatient clinics, and emergency rooms. Clinical nurses may rotate to different parts of a hospital or begin to acquire skills in one specialty, such as maternity nursing.

Charge Nurse: a registered nurse who has the skills and experience to supervise an entire hospital unit—for example, the hospital maternity ward.

Nurse Practitioner: a nurse who has completed a course of study at the graduate level, enabling him or her to perform as a primary care provider to patients. A primary care nurse provider can examine a patient and assess her health. This individual can take therapeutic action based on the established practices of the medical specialty.

Nurse Midwife: a nurse who has been certified for entry into practice according to the requirements of the American College of Nurse-Midwives and who practices nursing management of women throughout their uncomplicated pregnancies. When a pregnancy becomes high-risk, the nurse midwife may continue to provide part of the care in support of the maternal-fetal medicine specialist.

Perinatal Nurse Specialist: a nurse who has completed a course of study, usually at the graduate level, as preparation to provide highly skilled care to pregnant women.

Licensed Practical Nurse: a nurse who provides the technical supportive parts of nursing care.

Neonatal Nurse Specialist: a nurse who is a specialist in the nursing care of premature, small-for-gestational-age, and sick babies. This specialty requires knowledge and skills in the most advanced medical treatment techniques of intensive care.

13

*

Additional Team Members

The medical management of your bedrest pregnancy is truly a team effort. As your pregnancy progresses, you may receive supportive services from a physical therapist, an occupational therapist, a dietitian, and one or more social workers.

These health professionals work in departments of medical centers, are staff members of your doctor's practice group, or are themselves in private practice. Their offices may be located in the same building as your doctor or you may need to travel to another location to see them. If you are hospitalized, these individuals will visit you at your bedside.

Their services may consist of a one-time consultation or continue throughout your bedrest pregnancy. You should keep their names and telephone numbers handy at your bedside table. The medical fees charged by these health professionals are usually covered by medical insurance plans. Make sure that your doctor initiates the referral in writing and attaches a copy of this document to your claim forms.

Physical Therapist

In Chapter 4, "Physical Positions," you read about the proper steps to follow in pushing yourself up to a sitting position and getting out of bed. A physical therapist can teach you how to maneuver in your bed without increasing pressure on your abdominal muscles and without breath-holding. You can learn how to position yourself during your lying-down time and while performing specific exercises.

Wait a minute, you're thinking. Did I just read the word "exercise"? Yes, it is possible that you will be allowed to perform certain exercises during your bedrest weeks. The reason why you are first reading about a bedrest exercise program in this chapter is that this is a relatively new development in the field of high-risk pregnancy management.

Physical therapists have long recognized that people who are on restricted activity need specific exercise programs to minimize the negative effects of lying down. But the specific exercises that are consistently best for pregnancy bedresters are just emerging from clinical testing to wider acceptance: the members of the OB/GYN section of the American Physical Therapists Association are focusing their efforts on developing exercise programs for women experiencing routine and high-risk pregnancies.

The Physical Therapy Department of Hutzel Hospital, in Detroit, Michigan, has developed a general exercise and educational program that has been published as a three-part series in the professional journal *Clinical Management*. Similarly, the Physical Therapy Department at Mercy Medical Center, a hospital in suburban Minneapolis–St. Paul, has developed a series of exercises designed to maintain strength and flexibility when a person is restricted to bedrest. Its guidelines have been utilized by other medical clinics, including the Mork Women's Clinic of Anoka, Minnesota. The OB/GYN nurses and physical therapists of Lutheran Hospital in LaCrosse, Wisconsin, have also developed a program that is available to doctors and hospitals.

A physical therapist (P.T.) can teach you exercises in a hands-on fashion, helping you practice until you fully understand how you should feel when moving your arms and legs correctly. Follow-up monitoring of your exercise program may be conducted by your nurse. Your doctor or nurse will make this referral.

Occupational Therapist

In Chapters 6 and 7, "Setting Up Your Room" and "Setting Up Your Room for Children," you learned about the importance of keeping objects at your bedside within arm's reach. But constant reaching for objects while lying on your side or on a tilt can strain your neck, back, and arm muscles. You may even experience some eyestrain.

An occupational therapist (O.T.) can teach you how to modify your hand activities and perform low-resistance coordination work to minimize this strain. You learn how to accomplish the daily tasks of eating, reading, writing, using the telephone, and doing craftwork while maintaining your bedrest position. You will be shown how to slightly alter the angle of your hands, your shoulders, and your back to prevent stress to your muscles and spine.

Occupational therapist house calls are still very rare, but if you are hospitalized, an occupational therapist will visit you. Your first talk may concentrate on the mechanics of using your hospital bed, adjusting the room, and possibly suggestions for craft projects. Prior to your discharge, you will talk to the occupational therapist about the ways and means of setting up your bedrest room at home. If you remain hospitalized for an extended period of time, the occupational therapist will visit you every few days, encouraging you in your activities of daily living and modified self-care techniques. This medical team member is always a welcome visitor at your hospital bedside.

Registered Dietitian

In Chapter 16, "Managing Your Household," we recommend that you seek a referral from your doctor to a dietitian. A dietitian can provide you with a variety of meal plans that are tailored to your level of activity and specific medical condition. You may need a lower calorie intake each day but not know where to cut back in your diet. Only a registered dietitian can teach you how to structure your meals to provide all the nutrition you need with a reduced calorie level. A dietitian can also structure meals for you and your family that provide variety and nutrition and are relatively simple to prepare.

Social Workers

Two types of social workers may provide support to you and your family during your bedrest pregnancy. In the next chapter, you will read about many tough issues in seeking your medical entitlements. A social worker can provide you with concrete information about state and local government assistance programs as well as nonprofit groups who can help you. Social workers who specialize in identifying concrete medical services usually work in hospitals or outpatient clinics of regional medical centers. Your nurse or doctor will refer you to this social worker, who may visit you in the hospital, the outpatient clinic, or call you at your home.

A social worker is also a person to whom you can talk about your blue days and your fears. In the section called "Taking Stock of All the Changes" on pages 137–218, you will read about certain moments when your fears and your depression may feel overwhelming. Just as your doctor and nurse guide you through the medical management of your high-risk pregnancy, a social worker can guide you through the emotional stages of a bedrest pregnancy. Social workers who concentrate on therapeutic counseling work in outpatient clinics, hospitals, and in private practice. Again, your nurse or doctor can make the appropriate referral for you.

*

TEMPORARILY
REORGANIZING
YOUR LIFE

*

14

*

The Costs of
Bedrest

When you first decided to become or found out you were pregnant, you began to make plans for taking maternity leave, buying a layette, and even thinking about child care in the future. Now all the plans you started to make are changed. This pregnancy is going to have all sorts of costs, and it's difficult to figure out where to begin making a new budget.

There are no easy solutions to handling the various costs of a bedrest pregnancy. There are different kinds of expenses with different kinds of payments required. Sometimes problems are more manageable when they are separated into different categories. This chapter presents the categories of financial costs in a bedrest pregnancy.

Medical Costs—
Private Medical Insurance Plans

If you are currently employed or are covered under another family member's health plan, reread the benefits plan to figure out your medical entitlements. If the plan is yours, you are the subscriber. If you are listed on a medical plan, the family member who is paying for the plan is the subscriber. You are either a subscriber, a spouse (wife), or a dependent (member of the family).

All medical plans have a separate listing for the costs of a standard pregnancy. These costs include the delivery of the baby, including vaginal and Cesarean surgery. The cost of prenatal care given by your doctor is all or partially paid for by the plan. Hospitalization during labor and delivery and after the birth (postpartum) is also listed on the medical plan.

How does your bedrest pregnancy differ from the costs listed on your plan? First, you need more prenatal care—more visits to your doctor and, perhaps, home visits by a nurse. Second, you need more medical tests. Third, you may need surgery prior to the birth of your baby. Fourth, you may need to be hospitalized prior to the birth of your baby. Fifth, you need equipment to manage your bedrest at home.

To make this situation even more complicated, your doctor can't predict exactly what you are going to need as your pregnancy progresses. Once a specific medical complication is diagnosed, your doctor can begin a specific course of care, but how long you will be on bedrest, whether you need surgery, whether you need to be hospitalized, are day-to-day decisions.

During the first days of your pregnancy bedrest, contact the personnel office of the company (yours or your husband's) that handles the medical plan under which you are covered. Speak to the employee benefits specialist, who handles medical claims. Tell the specialist that your pregnancy has been diagnosed as high-risk and needs special medical management. The employee benefits specialist will have information for you and will also refer you to a claims counselor who represents the medical insurance carrier.

The medical insurance plan will pay for the costs of your bedrest pregnancy in two ways: 1) direct payment to your doctor or your hospital based on bills received; and/or 2) payment to you, after reviewing a paid bill submitted by you. In either case, a check is issued for a specific amount toward the service rendered, or a percentage of that bill (claim reimbursement).

You, the benefits specialist, the medical plan claims counselor, and your doctor's billing secretary (or the hospital billing office counselor for hospital bills) must all work together to keep the processing of your medical claims operating smoothly: You obtain medical claim reimbursement forms from the employee benefits specialist, fill out the forms at home, and bring them to your doctor's billing secretary at every appointment. Submit your claim forms to the hospital billing accounts office when you are hospitalized. Keep a list and photocopies of the claims you submit and check with the appropriate billing clerks every two weeks to find out if reimbursements have been received.

In your doctor's office, a billing clerk sends your claim reimbursement form to the medical insurance company. The clerk and the insurance claims counselor will talk to each other about the specifics of the claim.

The claims counselor and employee benefits specialist will be in contact to review the terms of the employer's plan that apply to you.

If you need specific medical supplies and equipment to manage your bedrest at home, you must get a written prescription from your doctor for this equipment in order to submit a medical claim. Ask your doctor to write these items on a claim reimbursement form or on a prescription slip and sign it at the bottom. Submit the claim form or prescription and your paid bill from the medical supply store to your medical plan company.

The Balance of the Medical Bill

After all the claims are filed and all the reimbursement checks are issued, there will still be a remaining balance that you owe for the bedrest pregnancy. You will owe money to your doctor and you will owe money to your hospital. It may take a few months for all your claim forms to be processed. By the time you receive your final bills, you will be back on your feet again, with a good idea of your family income and expenses. Both your doctor's billing clerk and the hospital's billing office counselor will work with you to set up a reasonable schedule of payments that will fit your new budget.

Medical Costs—
Without Private Medical Plan Coverage

If you are *not* covered by a medical insurance plan, the expenses of a high-risk pregnancy can be staggering. If your family income is above the government guidelines for the poverty level and you are not covered by an employer medical plan, you will find you are not eligible for many social services. Unfortunately, most social services programs apply only to families whose income and assets fall below a certain level.

As soon as possible, you need to be referred to a social worker who specializes in obtaining concrete medical and social services. You may need to be treated by specific perinatal medical centers and be hospitalized in certain hospitals in order to receive social services. (You may be comforted to know that many medical centers that accept social services patients are often the large regional centers that provide some of the most advanced care.)

You may also need to consider applying for a loan to cover your expenses. This is a tough decision to make, but there may be advantages to paying a loan rather than reducing your financial assets.

Filing Medical Deductions on Your
Income Tax

Medical costs and related expenses not covered by your medical plan or social services can be filed as medical deductions in your annual income tax return. You need to discuss with a certified public accountant your current financial situation and the best way to prepare for filing an itemized tax return that lists these medical expenses. Your accountant may suggest that taking a loan and then filing medical expenses may be a good way to manage your family budget.

If you are the subscriber to a medical plan or are filing a joint return with the subscriber, the medical premiums listed on the paycheck are also valid medical deductions.

The cost of child care during your bedrest and a homemaker to take care of your cooking and cleaning are usually not covered by your medical plan but are related expenses for the management of your pregnancy bedrest.

Keep complete and accurate lists of all the expenses related to your pregnancy and review them with the accountant. You need an expert in the field of tax accounting to review your total family income and expenses and advise you how best to prepare your income tax return.

What About Nonmedical Items?

The walkie-talkies, extra bedsheets, and flat-buttomed roaster pan you needed for eating were a great help but are not valid medical expenses for your medical plan or for your income tax return. This is one of the reasons we tried to provide lists of items to use and to wear that are inexpensive and can be used after you are back on your feet.

> I have some very special commuter cups on my dashboard. I remember taking them out to my car after my bedrest pregnancy and saying to them, "This is your new home." There's something special about watching my daughter sipping a drink from one of my cups on her way to ballet lessons.

The Cost of Not Working

The next chapter outlines how to apply for disability leave from your job.

If you are continuing to pay your company premiums for medical insurance or you are continuing coverage under another medical plan, most of the medical expenses will be reimbursed. But the change in your family income is going to mean a rejuggling of the budget. If your job income was paying for certain bills, your family budget may not be able to cover these payments.

Work out a revised budget that covers your basic needs and figure out what you could pay to each bill every month. Contact your creditors and explain your situation. Often they will agree to smaller payments for a period of time. State and local governments have financial counselors who can meet with your family to review your outstanding bills and talk directly to your creditors. These counselors may be able to adjust all payments, including utilities and mortgages, to fit your reduced monthly income. Don't wait until the creditors start to send you late notices. When you take the first steps, you have the best chance to work with your creditor in modifying a payment schedule.

Because you are not working, your family income may temporarily meet the eligibility requirements for certain government and social services assistance. As mentioned earlier, work with a social worker who specializes in obtaining government assistance.

Cooking Costs

You are going to eat about the same now as you have been eating throughout your pregnancy. With the tips in Chapter 16, "Managing Your Household," your family will eat just about the same way, too. You might want to purchase an electric slow cooker, a crockpot. Switching to paper plates and plastic utensils will add to your food budget.

Your family might eat take-out food more often, which will change your budget a bit. But many bedresters receive casseroles and cookies from friends and these gifts actually reduce their food costs.

Clothing Costs

You do fairly well in this category. You need only one to two pregnancy outfits for your doctor's appointments. In Chapter 10, "Your Wardrobe," the list of clothes you need is about the same as it would be if you were on your feet. You can continue to use after your pregnancy the T-shirts and sweat pants you now wear during the day.

Child Care Costs

The cost of caring for your children depends upon their ages. School-age children need help getting to and from school and outside activities. If you work out an arrangement with one mother, you could offer to pay her gas costs in exchange.

If your child is in a day-care center, continuing this arrangement may be still cheaper than letting the child stay at home with a paid caregiver.

If you have been taking care of your young child at home, you need to budget the cost of a caregiver for all or part of the day while you are restricted in your activities. You may be able to hire an individual who will care for your child and do some light housekeeping or the laundry.

Keep records of all child care expenses, including costs of a sitter when it is necessary to have this help in the evening. These are valid expenses to submit in your annual income tax return.

Cleaning Costs

The basic care of your home, both cleaning and cooking, is considered custodial care by medical plan companies. Custodial care is not reimbursed as a medical benefit. However, it may qualify as a valid tax deduction if it is properly documented by you and your doctor.

You will need to hire an individual to do specific cleaning chores in your home periodically. You can contact a cleaning service through your telephone directory or post a want ad at a local university, high school, or youth center.

The advantage of using a cleaning service is that the workers are insured, so breakage costs are covered as well as any pilferage losses. The service is then more expensive than hiring help directly. If you post your own ad and someone responds, be sure to get three or more references, preferably from teachers and youth counselors. You must pay the minimum hourly wage. If your budget allows you to spend twenty-five dollars every two weeks for cleaning, turn that into the number of hours at the minimum wage rate when you advertise.

Contact Costs

Your contact with the outside world will require a radio and a television set. You may need to budget for the cost of renting a television set in your bedroom.

If you have a VCR, you need to budget for the cost of renting videotapes. Library tapes have no rental fees. If you watch five or more tapes each week, the rental cost is going to begin to be noticeable in your budget. One bedrester had an interesting way of budgeting for rentals: she figured that she spent about six dollars per week on pantyhose when she went to work. Since she didn't need pantyhose while on bedrest, this money could be used to rent videotapes.

You may need to remember to budget for outside activities for your family. If they enjoy ice-skating or like going out to a movie with friends, it's important for them to continue even if you can't join them.

Crafts Costs

Chapter 17, "Expanding Your Horizons," has many ideas for activities to do during the day. Most activities need only a few items easily purchased in a supermarket, toy store, or craft outlet. For needle crafts, you need to budget for the cost of tools and kits. Save your receipts from all purchases in craft stores. Often, the craft store will give you a refund for unused or extra skeins of wool returned within a reasonable time period.

15

*

Your Job

If you are currently working at a paying job, the news that your pregnancy is high-risk and requires bedrest is a jolting, nasty surprise. As you read in Chapter 2, "Why Bedrest for My Pregnancy?" bedrest may be prescribed in low dosages, requiring a modification in daily activities, or it may be required full-strength, requiring that all active work be stopped immediately. Both situations present problems for the working woman.

Modifying Your Work Schedule

Pregnancy bedrest positioning may be advised as part of a plan to "take it easy." What does "taking it easy" mean to you when you are working full-time and managing your household? We recommend that you and your nurse and doctor carefully review your work schedule and your household chores. Use the bedrest checklist in Appendix 3 to help define your limitations specifically.

If possible, you may want to think about continuing to work on a part-time schedule. If your supervisor approves of this change, you will need to develop a workweek that is consistent with your restrictions. For example, working part of each day requires you to commute five days a week. Cutting back to three or two days reduces the stress of commuting.

Or you might be able to get yourself reassigned temporarily to an area of work that enables you to sit (and reduce your hours to a part-time schedule). Your job, especially if it is desk work, may be less physically exhausting than loading washing machines and cleaning floors at home. When you are working on a part-time basis, don't take on household chores to fill the rest of the day.

Reducing your work hours may affect your rate of leave accrual and benefits. Before you start a part-time schedule, carefully review these changes with the person in charge of employee benefits at your company.

Working on a part-time schedule may continue as long as your medical complication remains stable. As your pregnancy progresses, your limitations may increase, finally reaching a level at which you must stop work.

When You Stop Working

Many working women have traveled from their jobs to a midday doctor's appointment only to be advised to begin full-strength pregnancy bedrest immediately.

Even if you have already been cutting back on your work hours, you may feel conflicted. Perhaps you are expected back at your job for a meeting or need to finish a project. Do you return to finish out the day? Should you return to work and talk to your supervisor? Maybe if you stayed late today, you could clean up your work and start your bedrest tomorrow.

It's a lot easier to answer these questions if you look or feel sick. If your doctor had just put your leg or your arm in a plaster cast, you probably wouldn't return to finish your workday. If you had just learned you needed to have your appendix removed, you wouldn't postpone the surgery until after you had completed cleaning out your work area or shopped for the monthly groceries.

But, for most high-risk pregnancies, you don't feel pain, even during the medical examination. And when you look in the mirror, you don't look sick. Even when you are shown a medical problem, by use of medical equipment, or look at diagrams or models of your uterus, you simply don't feel too ill or weak to work.

Nevertheless, full-strength pregnancy bedrest for a high-risk pregnancy complication means that you are *immediately, temporarily disabled.* Those three words are what you must say to your supervisor, the personnel office, and/or coworkers. You are temporarily disabled and entitled to receive the same benefits of disability leave that any other employee in your company, male or female, receives for a broken leg, arm, accident, or operation.

Your Legal Rights

If you are working in a company that employs a minimum of fifteen employees, you have a federal law to protect you from discrimination based on your complicated pregnancy. The Pregnancy Discrimination Act (P.L. 55-555), passed in 1978, prohibits discrimination based on pregnancy, childbirth, or directly related medical conditions. You cannot be discriminated against in hiring, promotion, firing, seniority, and related personnel policies. Your pregnancy complication must be covered by your business's temporary disability policy or sick leave.

In addition, working in a company that employs a minimum of fifteen employees, you retain your right to a job at your company when you return from your extended leave. However, your company does have a right to reassign a coworker to your current job and offer you a comparable job when you return from your extended leave.

At present, forty-three states have passed similar laws that extend you state protection as well. Some states have passed pregnancy discrimination laws that extend protection to companies that employ less than fifteen employees. We recommend that you contact your state government department of labor to learn your legal rights for disability leave. Don't hesitate to call because you feel your question is unusual. Questions about pregnancy discrimination are among the most common inquiries these government offices receive each day.

If you learn that P.L. 55-555 and your state laws do not protect you in your current job, don't be discouraged. Follow the steps outlined in this chapter for leaving your job and applying for sick leave and extended leave. Use the words "disability leave" to describe your current situation. Your talks with your employer should follow the same lines as talking to a supervisor in a large company. Your calm, knowledgeable approach will encourage your employer to carefully consider your requests.

If you are not covered by federal and state laws and you cannot reach a reasonable agreement with your employer, you may be separated from your job. Immediately apply to your state department of labor for unemployment and disability benefits. You have a legal right to these benefits and you have paid taxes to provide for these government programs that you now need. When you apply for a job in the future, state specifically why you were separated.

At Your Doctor's Office

If you have just been told to start bedrest and have been given this book, turn to Chapter 3, "Immediate Arrangements."

The First Morning of Your Disability Leave

Whether you are lying on a hospital bed or lying on your own bed at home, the morning after your office appointment you're going to wake up a bit more ready to deal with the issues of your job.

Telephoning Your Supervisor

Think about what you want to say *before* you call. You may want to write a few phrases to keep in front of you while you talk. Again, you want to state that your doctor has diagnosed a medical complication that is a temporary disability. You need to begin a period of *disability leave* from your job. You will need to telephone the personnel office to arrange for your leave.

This is not a social call. Try not to explain all the details of your medical condition. Keep the conversation focused on your application for a leave from your job, and what work you were going to do today and can't. If you can't remember all your meetings or appointments, ask a coworker to flip through your weekly appointment book or read to you from your desk calendar.

State clearly that you want to work out all the issues of your leave from your job first, and then discuss the work you can no longer finish. Set a telephone appointment date and time, at least three working days from this day, to talk about your work.

Telephoning the Personnel Office

Your next telephone call will be easier. Company personnel offices or human resources departments, as many are now called, usually have one or more staff members who specialize in employee benefits. They will help you manage two major issues of your high-risk pregnancy: 1) your medical benefits, and 2) your leave from work. The procedure for applying for medical benefits is covered in the preceding chapter.

To begin your application for a leave from your job, your doctor must fill out your company's official "leave slip," stating the diagnosis of your medical complication and the nature of your restricted activity. The employee benefits specialist will mail this leave slip to you (with a set of medical claim forms), and will contact the payroll office to determine how much annual and sick leave you have earned as an employee.

Your company may require you to use your annual and sick leave as part of your disability leave. Your company may provide additional paid disability leave, or may continue you as an unpaid employee for the rest of your disability leave.

Your paychecks have included a stub that lists your gross pay and all the portions of money that you paid for a medical plan, insurance (both called "premiums"), and taxes. Your company also pays premiums for the enrollment of its employees in a medical plan, insurance, and government unemployment insurance. While you are on unpaid leave, your company will continue to pay its premiums to keep you enrolled for your medical plan, insurance, and certain other benefits. But, you, too, must continue to pay your medical and insurance premiums during your unpaid leave. The person handling employee benefits can check to see if these premiums change during your disability leave and unpaid leave. This is a cost you must plan for in your family budget.

It takes a while to review all of your payroll and personnel records. But, within a day or two, the employee benefits specialist will be able to tell you:

- how many paychecks you will be receiving, based on your annual and sick leave earned
- how long you are entitled to disability leave
- the amount and the method of continuing to pay for your medical and insurance premiums
- how your leave will change at the end of your pregnancy

If you have been picking up your paycheck at your job, try to arrange for these next paychecks to be directly deposited in your bank account. The employee benefits specialist will help you arrange for direct deposit of your paychecks.

You may not apply for unemployment insurance while you are on disability leave or an extended leave without pay from your job. Your company is still carrying you on their employment rolls even if you are not receiving a paycheck. You must leave your job in order to collect unemployment insurance. Remember that if you quit your job, you must pay for your medical costs yourself or with social services assistance. If you quit your job because of your pregnancy, your company does not have to rehire you when you are ready to return to work.

Your First Week of Disability Leave

In a few days, you will have a better idea of how your medical complication is going to be managed, you will have adjusted a bit to your bedrest positioning and restricted activities, and you will know how long and how much your disability leave is going to be.

Once these issues are settled, you will feel calmer about talking to your supervisor about your unfinished work.

Now is the moment to keep that telephone appointment. The purpose of this call is to close out your work. If you hold a desk job, your supervisor or someone he or she designates sits at your desk, calls you, and talks to you about all the papers on top and in the drawers. This may seem very difficult, because all employees have unfinished work and feel uncomfortable discussing it. But now is the best time to settle business. It is much better to keep this telephone appointment than for your supervisor and other workers to search through your desk to find a business letter or an invoice.

Should you try to finish some work at home? This question raises several issues: first, how can your company compensate or pay you for work you do at home? Can you work while you are on disability leave? Is this work stressful? Will you need to make telephone calls? Would it be more efficient for your company to let another person try to finish your work and then review the results with you? When you are trying to solve all the impossible tasks, will the work you do at home be of the same quality that you produced at your office?

It's difficult to let go of work you feel is your own and run the risk of someone else taking over your job. Becoming temporarily disabled and restricted in your activities means learning to accept that some of your work has to be done by others.

Is there any work that can be done at home while on bedrest? If you work in sales or at a service center, your work will be picked up by coworkers immediately. Some customer-service jobs require you to keep your customer list handy and do telephone contacts. Still, in these jobs, you need access to the inventory data of your company, as well as clerical help. Secretarial work and clerical work can be performed temporarily at work by coworkers, or by a temporary service. Writing jobs would seem to be accomplished easily at home, but writing requires concentration and you may discover you are not able to concentrate fully on your job during your high-risk pregnancy. If you work as a computer programmer or analyst or your work requires a computer terminal, you may consider placing a keyboard on your bed and trying to complete some projects. The most important point in considering working at home is that you will not be able to work an eight-hour day. Your goals should be scaled down to what you are able to do for a few hours each day.

Your Second Week of Disability Leave

As you adjust to the rhythm of your restricted daily schedule, you may still miss the rushing around of going to work. From your window, you can hear the sounds of cars pulling out of driveways on the way to work and to drop off schoolchildren. You wake up with the energy to start a workday and you think of your office where your friends are laughing over their coffee mugs. Your coffee mug is still at work, along with all the photos and personal items you like to have around you.

A coworker may offer to bring your personal items to you, but carefully think through this offer before agreeing. First, you are on temporary disability leave and your personal items on your desk or hanging near your work area symbolize your intention to return to work. Second, even if you do want your personal items at home during your leave, do you want your colleagues to visit you at home while you are on bedrest? If not, you might ask a member of your family to visit your office briefly to retrieve your personal items.

During this second week, your office and coworkers are adjusting to working without you. This is the time to begin calling your workplace once a week to keep in touch about what is happening. If you keep in touch, you may be kept in mind for future projects, and your colleagues may gain added respect for you in the way you are able to take charge of a temporary situation that might overwhelm others.

Keep in touch with a coworker you already trust. You need to know about new employees, new policies, and new projects for your company. You can continue to be part of the information network at your job.

You might enjoy receiving phone calls from the office—being called for advice or information makes you feel a part of the action. But you might find that such unexpected phone calls are interfering with your emerging bedrest schedule. If so, try to schedule an office hour in your daily routine. A telephone answering machine can help enforce the times when you do not want to be disturbed.

If you are sensing difficulties with your supervisor, it may not be your disability leave but your changing role as a working mother that is the source of the problem. Often a working woman must discuss with her supervisor the details of her changing lifestyle as her pregnancy progresses. Because you are not at the office, you are unable to meet these issues together face to face. Your supervisor may also hesitate to bring up such issues because of your unstable medical condition.

You may also find during these weeks that some of your coworkers are not as friendly as you might have expected. Your high-risk pregnancy may be intensifying some hidden anxieties for them. Chapter 26, "Your Friends," addresses this issue.

Now My Plans for Maternity Leave Are Completely Ruined

When you became pregnant, you began to make plans for when you would stop working, how long you would remain at home with your baby, and if you would like to return to work, perhaps returning to a different work schedule.

Bedrest makes one change in your pregnancy plans: the date you stop working temporarily. You may have planned on earning annual leave and sick leave right up to your due date and then using this accumulated leave after your baby's birth. The date you begin bedrest is the date you begin to use all the annual and sick leave you had previously earned. During your disability leave, you do *not* continue to earn annual and sick leave.

Also, after your pregnancy, if your baby needs medical monitoring in the hospital, and you are returning to your job, you may need additional leave from work and a modified work schedule to enable you to be with your baby during each day.

A high-risk pregnancy requiring temporary disability leave does not change who you are as an expectant mother. Every pregnant woman makes plans for how she will handle motherhood and her job. And every woman who becomes a mother, no matter how uneventful her pregnancy, will discover that becoming a mother changes her in ways she can't anticipate. Books and magazine articles appear every month about the ways women balance their role as parents with their economic needs and personal career goals.

When Disability Leave Becomes Maternity Leave

When you are no longer pregnant, your disability leave from work may convert to maternity leave (sometimes called "parental leave"). The company policy for maternity or parental leave applies to the time just before delivery and a period of time afterward. Disability leave for a medical complication stops just before you enter the labor and delivery suite. Maternity leave then begins with a live birth.

If your pregnancy ends without a live birth, you are entitled to *continue your disability leave* until you are completely recovered from the effects of the medical complication. Your doctor should specify in writing the reasons for extending your disability leave and this should be attached to your correspondence to the personnel office.

16

*

Managing Your Household

Cooking and cleaning are the two major parts of managing your household, and both will be off-limits for you during your bedrest pregnancy. Perhaps bedresters worry the most about their household because cleaning and cooking were the simple tasks they had to do each day before their pregnancies were diagnosed as high-risk and requiring restricted activity. They cleaned the bathroom sink when it needed a scrub; did the laundry, daily and weekly; loaded the dishwasher; and baked a batch of brownies for a treat. Now, they worry, the home will just get dirtier and the leftovers will turn to mold in the refrigerator.

Worrying about cooking and cleaning can lead to the "just-a-few-minutes" behavior. The second trip to the bathroom, a second look at that bathroom sink, and you're reaching for the cleanser and sponge for a few minutes' wipe-up. While you're holding the cleanser, why not scrub off the ring in the bathtub? How long can it take to stir chocolate pudding in a saucepan, the kind your child really misses? It only takes four minutes to unload a dishwasher, and then the dishes will be in the right cabinets. How difficult is it to hang a few towels?

My helper once opened the living-room window on a ninety-degree day and departed. I had to decide whether to air-condition the entire state or take a walk to the living room. I decided to stay in bed because I thought I knew myself too well. I was convinced that once I started to get up for any reason other than the bathroom and the doctor's visits, it would become impossible to keep from popping up all day.

Every one of us has been tempted to take "just a few minutes," to do some household task during our bedrest. And, yes, a few times we caught ourselves doing something beyond our specified limits. We felt guilty, frustrated, and angry.

Remember that part of the temptation to straighten up a room or clean out the refrigerator is boredom. If you have nothing to do, there's always housework. So the first trick in managing your household while you are restricted is to plan your schedule to minimize your boredom. The next chapter is crammed with ideas.

Cooking

How do I manage the cooking for myself and my family?

First, let's concentrate on you. You need to continue to eat a good basic pregnancy diet that supplies the right amount of calories over a twenty-four-hour period. You may have already received pamphlets about pregnancy care that contained lists of foods for a nutritious diet. Pregnancy diets consist of three regularly spaced meals and two snacks each day.

Your pregnancy diet plan may need to be modified based on your specific medical complications *and* your restricted activity. We urge you to talk to your doctor about your current diet plan and work closely with your nurse or, if you are referred, with a registered dietitian. These health professionals will help you create a diet plan that provides the nutrition you and your baby need, with the right amount of calories per day for you. Don't try to change your diet yourself; seek the advice of your doctor and the other health professionals.

When I became a diet-managed diabetic patient, the hospital dietitian created a meal plan that was completely different from what I had been eating at home, on bedrest. It was so much more food! But in just a few days I felt a lot better. My husband learned to measure the correct amounts of juice and bought a food scale to weigh my portions. The dietitian gave us complete lists of foods and sample menus that were easy to prepare.

Chapter 6, "Setting Up Your Room," has tips for eating while sitting up in bed or remaining in your bedrest position.

Breakfast

Start your day with breakfast in bed. A family member can make your meal while making his or her own; if you can't eat in the same room, at least you can be eating at the same time.

How would you eat a breakfast of juice, hot tea or coffee, cereal, and buttered toast? Carefully! Toast should be buttered before you receive it, cereal should be in a larger bowl than you usually need, and the juice and hot drink should be in plastic commuter cups with lids.

Remember to keep your plastic flexi-straws handy for drinking. When you begin to eat, prop one arm under your head for support or set up several extra pillows to raise your head slightly. Then, keep your tray close. You may not feel very elegant eating this way, but your immediate goal during meals is to prevent a sticky, gooey spill on your clothes or bedsheet.

Lunches

It's easier to prepare and eat a cold lunch—a daily picnic in bed. When family members are preparing their lunches for work and for school, they can pack a lunch for you in a picnic cooler. That cooler is placed next to your bed. You should also have two Thermos bottles nearby: hot and cold water handy for drinks during the day.

Would you like a turkey sandwich or last night's meatballs in tomato sauce on a roll? Both sound good. But one requires more skill in eating in bed. Stick to finger foods, such as wedges of cheese, celery and carrot sticks, apples, and breadsticks, until you become skilled in eating while lying on your side. Sip your soup from a cup with a drinking lid. Eat your peas with a spoon. When you prepare yourself for a meal, clean your hands with a cleansing wipe, and tuck a dish towel into your neckline to cover your front. Reusable dish towels are much cheaper in the long run than paper disposables.

Snacks

A pregnancy snack can be another, smaller sandwich and fruit. Keep your snacks in your cooler, too.

Supper

Supper is the key meal for you and your family. If you are allowed to join your family at the table, *be the last to arrive and the first to leave.* Sitting with them is not the same as serving them or cleaning up afterward.

It's not what you and your family are planning to eat but how long it takes to cook that can cause the most problems. One of the ways to have a hot meal ready for all of you is to use an electric slow cooker: a crockpot. A family member can fill the crockpot with meat and vegetables early in the morning, during breakfast preparations, and it will cook all day, making a piping hot meal by suppertime. All your family has to do is prepare a salad and a dessert. If you already have a microwave oven, you know that it can heat food and cook meals quickly. Your family can cook and freeze several meals in advance, then defrost and heat each meal in the evening.

Cooking casseroles, meat loaves, and stews once a week and

storing them in the freezer is an excellent way to minimize cooking in the evening. A friend or relative who enjoys cooking can make and freeze meals and then bring them to your freezer. Your family can supply the food or reimburse her (or him) later.

Vegetables and fruits can be washed, chopped, and bagged every few days. Then your family can reach for these bags to create salads and portion vegetables for steaming or boiling. Steaming and boiling food should be done by an older family member, not a young child.

If your family is not doing well with dishwashing, they may be better off with a stack of paper plates and plastic utensils for this temporary period. A spongeable plastic tablecloth will make table cleanups faster and easier, too.

If you are eating your supper in bed, try to arrange for the family to join you for all or part of their meal. They can eat on snack tables or use one card table. Even if you all just eat and watch the evening news, it's nice to be together for supper.

Planning the Family Meals

If you have been the family shopper, other members of your family are going to be going to the supermarket, often with interesting results:

> When my husband learned that I would need to spend most of my days off my feet for two weeks, he immediately went to the supermarket and bought $292 worth of groceries.

You can manage the family food budget by preparing specific shopping lists and planning complete meals. Make sure that there is a backup of frozen dinners, for situations in which the first meal planned backfires. Also, try to budget for at least one take-out meal every week. It can be pizza, tacos, fried chicken, or an Asian dish. If your family shops in the evening, they might enjoy eating out first. You can arrange your sitting-up privileges to supervise the unloading of the groceries.

If your family likes your cooking and baking, their own efforts will probably not taste as good or as familiar. If you like baking brownies from scratch and your family likes licking the bowl, let them experiment with a brownie mix. They may prefer your version but they will have the enjoyment of baking. Sometimes a family let loose in a kitchen can produce amazing results. One father was able to cook an entire Thanksgiving Day dinner without ever having cooked a full course dinner in his life. Another man discovered he enjoyed preparing salads. Children can make sandwiches they would never eat if you made them. All these good habits should be praised and encouraged to continue after you are back on your feet again.

Cleaning

How do I keep my home clean?

Our first answer to this question is, "You don't." The vacuuming, dusting, scrubbing, and clothes washing have to be done by others. Even if you have some sitting-up and standing privileges during the day, housework is rough work. Talk to your doctor or nurse about the dos and don'ts of housework. Don't assume that because they didn't talk about cleaning, you can continue these tasks.

Managing your cleaning presents different problems than managing your cooking needs. Food preparation is essentially an enjoyable activity. Shopping for food has interesting moments; sometimes your family returns with a few items they'd like to try. Most family members will pitch in for meal preparation. Your friends and neighbors will make casseroles or baked goods for you and your family because it's a nice way to help.

Cleaning your home is as necessary as clipping your toenails and just about as exciting. Routine maintenance of your home is a set of chores. Your family complained about them and did them halfheartedly before you became pregnant; they won't stop complaining now. When your friend offers to cook a casserole, you wouldn't say to her, "Thanks, but our freezer is filled this week. By the way, do you think you could come over to clean my bathroom?"

So how do these chores get done? First, figure out what really needs to be cleaned. Get out your lap desk and make a list of all the rooms in your home and the chores that need to be done to keep each area clean. Then, start crossing out every chore that isn't absolutely necessary. For example, cleaning the venetian blinds can wait for a while. If you have been picking up after the family in the different rooms, think about bringing baskets into different areas to store toys and papers. Knickknacks could be temporarily packed away, couches and chairs covered with throws to protect them from spills and dirty shoes.

Once you have a good working list, have a straightforward talk with your family about what they can and can't do. Remember that they are doing the cooking and shopping now as well as many errands you used to do. You need to know who is able to clean the bedrooms, bathroom, and kitchen. Laundry is described below. When you have identified what your family can reasonably do, you will still have a list of routine chores that need to be done every week or every other week. You're going to need help and you should think about paying a house cleaner to do a full day of these chores every other week. If you need to be on bedrest for six weeks, that means hiring a house cleaner for three full days.

The ways and means to hire a house cleaner are described in Chapter 14, "The Costs of Bedrest." Here, we will repeat that it is not necessary to hire professional janitorial services. A student at a local college or high school has the strength, the time, and the need for extra money.

When is the best time to clean your home? One family arranged for a cleaner to come when they took the bedrest mom to her doctor's appointment. They all enjoyed coming home to a clean house. A weekend morning may be the best time for your part-time helper. When your room is being cleaned, move yourself to another area of the home. This can be your time for a shower or you can position yourself for a while on the living-room couch. Some of us arranged for the cleaning day to be a day or two before some friends were scheduled to visit.

One of the interesting discoveries of being at home all day is that you can finally wait for the repairman. "Sure," you say to the dispatcher, "I'm home today. All day." But being the only person at home means getting up to answer the door and being available for questions while the repair is being performed. You may be tempted to sit or stand by the plumber while the toilet is dismantled . . . or stand near your beloved dishwasher whose bottom fell out. A better idea is to explain to the dispatcher your current medical situation and try to arrange for a service appointment when your family is available.

After weeks of bedrest, no matter how carefully your family and house cleaner have worked, the home may need some intensive cleaning. Many pregnant women have suddenly had the urge to clean the oven or scrub the floor just before they went into labor. As you approach your due date, you may get the same urge. Channel your energy into arranging for a janitorial service to perform a ceiling-to-floor cleaning of your home, right after the baby is born and you're still in the hospital. It's better to bring your baby from the hospital to a clean house than to walk through the door and begin the cleaning yourself.

Laundry

The most efficient way to manage the family laundry is to schedule a once-a-week washing day. Washing clothes is really a series of hand motions: tossing the dirty stuff into different mounds, tossing the laundry into the machine, hanging up some laundry, loading the clothes dryer for other items, resorting and folding, and putting away. The more hands, the easier the work. Your participation is limited to offering your advice on how a garment should be washed. The other tasks are too strenuous. When your children's clothes are clean, you can save some time during the week by having your family assemble seven hangers of complete outfits.

Although figure 2 on page 21 shows an ironing board next to the pregnancy bedrester, we don't recommend trying to iron clothes while in bed. It is just plain unsafe. A family member will iron or learn to iron or you need to pay for ironing. This is the time to send men's shirts to a professional laundry. Now, the author who loves to iron wrote this paragraph. The other author hates the idea of ironing and gently suggests that many clothes items dry practically wrinkle-free and the family members might not mind a few wrinkles.

You can sort socks. You can also do a lot of mending. Repairing loose hems, sewing back buttons, and refitting elastic into waistbands will help maintain the family wardrobe.

17

*

Expanding Your
Horizons

How often have you said to yourself, "If only I had the time . . ."?
Now, for better or for worse, you have a lot of time each day, while
you are lying down, to do something other than household chores
and office work.

For the first day or two, it may take all your efforts just to learn
to remain lying down. You'll watch a lot of television and start to
read. Most bedresters read a lot of books, especially during the first
week. You have a lot of planning to do in the first weeks, creating a
new schedule for yourself, applying for medical benefits, and if you
were working, straightening out your disability leave. But as your
schedule takes shape, you're going to begin to wonder what else
you can do during the time between doctor appointments.

This is an idea list to inspire you. You couldn't possibly do every
activity in this chapter in one pregnancy. Every idea was suggested
or tested by a bedrester. Reread this chapter from time to time,
because your interests and attention span will change as your
pregnancy progresses. At certain times, you'll want a quick fix to
perk up your day; another week you might feel the urge to start a

longer project. We've even included a section entitled "Creative Television," because watching programs or videotapes is an activity that can help you cope with long periods of lying down.

READING

Phone your local library to arrange for special services such as deliveries for the homebound of books, book tapes, and even videotapes. Your librarian can prepare a set of books by one author or about one topic, ready for a friend to check out for you.

- Read every book by an author: every spy novel, every romance.
- Read every book in a series, fiction and nonfiction.
- If you like mystery novels, switch to science fiction.
- Read biographies of great people and famous villains.
- Read military history books if you want to avoid any mention of marriage, children, and pregnancy. If military history bores you, read it before your afternoon nap.
- Read books that will help you in your career.
- Read a road atlas: a magazinelike book of every state in our country or every country in the world. Take a mental vacation— plotting a trip across the west on Route 66, or figuring out how long it would take to drive to Orlando, Florida. Trace the names of towns across our country as the land was gradually settled.
- Reread your old textbooks. Remember how to do geometry? Or borrow your children's textbooks.
- Read all the sections of the newspaper. Get a different newspaper delivered. Or ask your friends to recycle their newspapers and magazines at your home.
- Subscribe to newsletters published by associations.
- Read recipe books.
- If you want to, read books about pregnancy.
- Read joke books. Learn knock-knock jokes, elephant jokes. Or read cartoon books.

RECEIVING MAIL

Receiving mail is a pleasure during bedrest. After a few days, even junk mail is going to look good to you.

• Send for every catalogue that advertises. You may find items you need during your bedrest and later on when you won't have time to shop either! One mail order house may sell its list to other companies so sending for one catalogue may result in receiving five others.
• Send for travel brochures, often advertised in the Sunday travel sections of newspapers.
• Write to consulates of foreign countries for pamphlets.
• Write to the local Chambers of Commerce for information about a town or city you'd like to visit. You might become interested in a town after "traveling" to it using your road atlas.

SENDING MAIL

• Enter every contest that is advertised in magazines and appears on cereal boxes and can labels.
• Write letters to editors in newspapers and magazines.
• Write to someone you don't know. For example, the armed forces has lists of men and women who have no one to write to and would like to receive letters.
• Address envelopes for a local charity, political group, PTA, or your church.

NEEDLE CRAFTS

A craft project keeps your hands active and gives your eyes a different focus point than the book or the television screen. You also get to enjoy what you have made:

My doctor appointments were once a week. As soon as I returned from a "good appointment," I started a new counted cross-stitch project and pushed myself to complete the picture by the next trip to the doctor. During one visit, my doctor asked me if I was spending all of my days in bed. I took out my just-completed project and said, "You know, I started this just after the last appointment and it's impossible to complete unless I spend *all* my time stitching!" After that, every appointment began with a display of the counted cross-stitch project I had completed during the week.

- Knitting: Your arms may feel strained when you use straight needles. If your knitting style is "European," try to learn the "American" style. Or use a circular needle, a long piece of plastic with pointed ends.
- Crocheting: Easier than knitting, especially if you are right-handed and lying on your left side. You can do a variety of quick items and even take out your old unfinished afghan quilt.
- Hooking a rug: Latch-hook rugs are surprisingly easy to make. You can loop the wool by hand or with a special inexpensive hook. There are kits of wall hangings, in all sizes.
- Embroidery: A tablecloth and napkins is a nice project.
- Stitchery: Most kits include clear directions for the different stitches. Investing in a small hoop for holding the material will be easier on your arms and hands. Use the metal frame from a large cosmetic mirror to hold the hoop on an angle.
- Knitting knobby work: Did you ever make a long tube of knitting from a cylinder with pegs on the top? This funny little device is inexpensive and you can use different materials to create belts, placemats, even berets.
- Macrame: You can make jewelry, wall hangings, and hangers for planters.
- Beadwork: You need to keep the beads in containers or else you'll feel like the princess and the pea. You can make bracelets, necklaces, even decorate clothes.

CUT-AND-PASTE CRAFTS

• Make birthday cards, holiday cards, your own stationery and postcards.
• Have your family bring you all the envelopes of photographs you never mounted and make albums.
• Start a cut-and-assembly kit. You can make entire bridges, skyscrapers, and dioramas.
• Has anyone actually tried the famous ship-in-the-bottle?
• Teach yourself origami, the art of paper-folding. Origami animals make beautiful holiday ornaments or mobiles.
• Make a cardboard scrapbook for your younger children.
• Make paper chains.
• Make a collage of wrapping paper from your baby gifts.

A *quick tip*: use glue sticks instead of pots of glue.

CLAY CRAFTS

• Kneading and molding clay is good exercise for your arms. Start with playdough (a mixture of salt, flour, and water) for inexpensive fun, then move up to air-dried modeling clay.
• Hobby and art supply stores have different ceramic clays that can be molded into jewelry and art objects.
• Create a suncatcher for your window. Hobby stores have kits that include a metal frame and packets of plastic granules. An aluminum foil-lined pie tin holds the metal frame and you spoon in the granules. (This is a family project for older children who are no longer putting their fingers in their mouths.) The granules and metal frame are baked in an oven, and the result resembles stained glass.

Another *quick tip*: keep a container of cleansing wipes nearby.

PENCIL AND PAINTBRUSH ART

• Use an inexpensive tray of water paints and paint a watercolor.
• Learn to draw. Your librarian can find an art textbook for you.

- Use pencils, typing paper, and erasers. Borrow your children's crayons or colored pencils.
- Use tracing paper on newspaper pictures or photographs.
- Try a paint or colored-pencil-by-number kit.
- Practice calligraphy.

> I'm left-handed, so lying on my left side made writing impossible. I decided to practice writing with my right hand, and in about a week my new writing was readable!

Third tip: for all wet work, put a plastic garbage bag on your lap tray and a second bag underneath you on the mattress.

GARDENING

- Did you ever grow a sweet potato vine? Three toothpicks will hold the sweet potato suspended in a cup of water.
- Start avocado plants from the large seeds.
- Prepare your summer gardening by setting up flats of seedlings.

These projects are wonderful to do with your children. Pick a seed that will have a growth pattern that approximates the length of your bedrest time. Then both you and your plants will be ready for "transplanting" at just about the same time!

LISTENING

- If you usually listen to country and western music, try tuning the radio dial to classical music, jazz, or rock.
- If you have a cassette tape player, listen to books on tape. Libraries have many tapes you can borrow, ranging from children's stories to current best sellers. Many famous movie stars are recording book tapes now.
- The old-time radio shows can be very enjoyable. You can listen to radio mysteries, comedies, even soap operas. Some of the current television soap operas started on radio. Children will enjoy these programs, too.
- Listen to the current radio talk shows.

TALKING

- Read and talk through a play. Memorize some lines and recite with feeling. You can play-act with your children. They can figure out how to make sound effects from listening to old radio show tapes.
- Learn a new language. Rent or borrow language tapes from the library. Certain travel stores rent or sell language tapes, too.
- Read about the art of ventriloquism and practice it.

PLAY A MUSICAL INSTRUMENT

- Yes, lying on your side, even lying on a tilt, you can play an electronic keyboard, xylophone, or a ukelele.
- You are never too old to learn to read music notes. With a basic music theory book, and an electronic keyboard, you will surprise yourself and your family.

SPECTATOR SPORTS

- Read about a particular sport and follow it in the news, the sports page, and television events.
- Rent exercise tapes and how-to educational tapes for specific sports. Develop your personal exercise plan for after your pregnancy when you are on your feet again.

CREATIVE TELEVISION

- If you like watching movies and other programs on television, try to budget for buying or renting a VCR, if you don't own one already.
- Most video stores can send you their lists of tapes. And your library will have books written about classic movies and television programs. You can develop a list of movies to see and match them to what is available in stores and libraries.
- Scan those video lists, library lists, and television listings for Alfred Hitchcock's movie, *Rear Window.* The key character has

broken his leg and spends his days looking out his window. He manages to witness a murder and solve a mystery.

- Record a full week of programs you missed while watching other channels. Play back these programs at a time convenient for you.
- Find a friend who enjoys watching the same television program that you do and talk by telephone while you both watch it. Watch game shows. You can guess along with the contestants. Several game shows have gadgets that enable you to play at the same time.
- While you watch one news program, record the other channel's news show. Then compare how the two programs handled the same story.

There are some days when you feel blue and depressed. Often you are experiencing the normal hormonal changes of pregnancy. But lying in bed for your medical complication just exaggerates your feelings. On these days, try using your television and video tapes to pick up your spirits. Tune in on every classic situation comedy, especially reruns of "I Love Lucy." Rent funny movies. One funny tape to try is *Ten from Your Show of Shows*. If the video store has some silent classics, try renting the Keystone Cops comedies.

DAYDREAM

Close your eyes and imagine a favorite street, restaurant, movie theater, department store, or park. Think about what you would do in each place. Plan how to get there, what you would wear, and imagine the sounds of each place. Daydreaming is total concentration and a way to temporarily experience being out of your bed.

EXPANDING YOUR HORIZONS WITH YOUR CHILD

The first time we wrote this chapter, we wrote a separate list of children's activities. Then we realized that almost all of these activities were identical to the activities we had recommended for you to do.

So, now we recommend that you find a craft or a project that you really enjoy doing and *share your enjoyment with your child.*

For example, if you have begun to enjoy drawing, give your child crayons and paper and draw together. If you are coloring by number, have your young child pick out the numbers and help you find the correct pencil. Teach your child to make a playdough bowl. Introduce your child to "Lucy." Teach your child to use a knitting knobby. Or teach your child how to do geometry problems. You can be the cutter for a diorama, and your child can position the piece on the building or bridge.

When your child sees you experimenting with an electronic keyboard or practicing your handwriting, she will copy your efforts. You might develop some special phrases in French with each other. If your teenager sees you struggling with a math problem, she might explain how to do it. Or your teenager might, just might, ask for your help in completing her homework!

When your child hears your laughter during a movie, watches your frustration in figuring out a stitch, or admires your skill in making a bird from a piece of paper, he sees and hears the familiar qualities of his mother. That's the most important message you can convey to your child during this bedrest time: that even though you're lying down for periods of time, you are still the same old Mom, the parent he loves.

18

*

Setting Up to Entertain

Living in southern California aboard a forty-two-foot sailboat, I survived four months of bedrest. Between the sound
of seagulls, salt air, and the lapping of the waves against the
boat, I lay in a special hammock hung between two masts.
Each day I passed the time waiting for my husband and son
to come home. Sometimes we would invite a crew to come
aboard and sail the boat around the Los Angeles harbor.
When that grew boring, we sailed across the open sea to
Catalina Island. It was truly an experience I will never
forget and today I enjoy my daughter and her love for
the sea.

Wow! Well, even if you aren't spending your bedrest on a sailboat,
you can still entertain yourself and visitors throughout your bedrest
pregnancy.

*First, discuss with your doctor and your nurse how often you
can have visitors to your home.* You already have specific privileges
for standing up, sitting, and showers. You may have to combine

113

your weekly allotment of "up" time with visits. You may be limited to half-hour visits, once a week, or be advised to spend an evening with friends every two weeks.

Once your limits have been set, recognize that within these limits, you may tire during a visit. When you make arrangements for friends to visit, pencil in extra rest time prior to their visit, and make the next day a quiet one. The more friends, the faster you will tire. So even if your doctor or nurse hasn't specified a visitor limit, try to keep the number to a minimum.

Choose the best area in your home to entertain friends. For example, you may temporarily set yourself up on the living-room couch and use the coffee table as your side table. If moving from your bed is not possible, limit your visitors to the number of comfortable places to sit in your room (no visitors on the bed, please). Folding snack tables or a card table can be set up nearby where you are lying down to put food, a board game, and drinks.

Dress for entertaining. Change into your daywear, even if your friends are coming over later in the evening. Some makeup, nail polish, a dab of perfume, and you look like yourself. If you remain in a nightgown looking tired and disheveled, you're encouraging your friends to make a sick call.

Pick an activity that focuses your family and friends on something other than you. Even if you can't actively participate, you're part of the conversation and the laughter. Here are some specific examples:

1. Your friends bring over a delicious home-cooked meal. It's a welcome treat for your family. If you are on a restricted diet, let your friends cook for your family and themselves, then eat your food with them.
2. Your friends bring over a pizza, take-out food, a picnic supper, or a restaurant meal. See item 1 above.
3. Your friends come over for a shorter evening of dessert and coffee. They bring a cake or you arrange for cakes and pastries from a local bakery. Coffee or tea is made in the kitchen and set up on the card table.
4. Your friends come over and play bridge, canasta, poker, or Old

Maid. Or they bring a board game like Trivial Pursuit or Othello. You can easily participate in most games while lying down. For example, you can roll dice in your bed and let a friend move a piece for you.

5. Your friends rent their favorite movie. Everyone munches on popcorn. Make sure your friends can see the screen clearly.
6. You and your friends form a book club to talk about a best seller or an old classic.
7. Your friends come over and help decorate your home for the holidays or have a gift-wrapping party to help you prepare presents for a family celebration.
8. Your friends and your family go out for a while—to a movie or to a restaurant. They all return for dessert and a short visit. This enables your family to relax and you can be part of the evening, too. Do this at least once during your bedrest time.

After several weeks of having friends over, I really began to enjoy Saturday evenings and I went ahead and scheduled the next two months. My husband realized that I had invited people to our home for the two weeks following my due date!

As your pregnancy progresses, your visitor privileges may be more restricted. Try switching to telephone calls. Chatting with a friend may be better than a brief visit that will feel more like a sick call.

Last, but not least, it is normal to feel tired after a visit. But if you are still feeling tired the day after a visit, even after a night's sleep and a nap, you probably overdid it. Make your next visit a shorter one and make the activity less active. For example, if you played a board game, you may want to switch to watching a movie.

*

BEDREST AWAY
FROM HOME

*

19

*

Short-term
Hospitalization

When I went to see my doctor at sixteen weeks, I felt
pleased with myself—past the first trimester, finished with
most of the fatigue and nausea, starting to look pregnant.
Before I knew it, I was down the hall from the examination
room, checking into the hospital for surgery, phoning my
husband and calling the sitter to say I wasn't coming home. I
was panicked. A kindly volunteer asked me if I was okay.
I said I was all right because I feared I would fall apart if I
started to really express how I felt. I couldn't seem to put on
my hospital gown and become a patient. I didn't want to lie
in the bed and wait for the doctors to come.

The very words, "I need to admit you to the hospital," are enough
to set your heart racing and weaken your knees. Ask any pregnant
woman what her doctor said *after* those first eight words, and she'll
usually say, "I can't remember what happened, it all became a
blur."

If you have just been told that you are being admitted to the hospital and you have been given this book, Chapter 3 can help you start to make immediate arrangements.

If you are reading this book after being admitted to the hospital, you've picked the right chapter to start!

Checking In

Your trip to the hospital was quick and quiet. All during this ride you kept saying to yourself:

> The doctor has found a problem. . . . I am going to the hospital because I have a problem. . . . The doctor found the problem in time. I hope he found the problem in time. . . . Going to the hospital is good . . . good. . . .

You needed to keep saying this to yourself because, at the same time you were thinking:

> Oh, no. I am going to be in a hospital room, lying on a hospital bed, wearing a hospital gown, and nurses and doctors are going to do things to me.

For many women, their first hospital experience in their entire life is being admitted to a hospital for the birth of their first child. Even for this happy event, the idea of entering a hospital, being admitted as a patient, being a patient, is a bit scary.

Perhaps that's why we tell funny stories about women and men who are trying to get to a hospital in time to have their baby. The father is always confused and the mother is always peaceful and calm as she is wheeled through the doors to the maternity ward. We know, also, that these silly stereotypes help us laugh at a situation that is not at all funny. Every pregnant woman admitted to a hospital tries to balance her relief at being safe with her fear of becoming a patient.

Your first impression of your hospital may not have calmed your fears. The admissions area may have been noisy and crowded, you may think you were admitted too slowly or you were rushed and felt confused. You may have seen sick and injured people and medical equipment. The beeping of the medical machines, the crying, and even the chatter of the nurses and doctors seemed too loud and upsetting.

Your first hour in your hospital room was very hectic; several young doctors asked you the same questions, nurses came in and out of the room, took your blood pressure from a piece of equipment on the wall, and showed you how to press a button on your bed to signal for help. All around you, decisions were being made about how to stabilize your medical condition.

Then, suddenly, you were lying in a bed, just the way you pictured it, and the hospital room seemed too quiet and still. Maybe you heard voices outside your room, but you couldn't understand the words. You began to be anxious and tense—how long have you really been here?

All people admitted to hospitals experience these same feelings. During the first hours, it's very common for new patients to lose track of time, be unable to concentrate very well, or become sensitive to noises outside in the hospital hall. Many people have daydreams, and many have felt an arm or a leg fall asleep. Talk to your nurse about these feelings. Talking will make you feel better. These new-patient feelings will gradually change.

Here is a short list of items that will help you orient yourself to being in a hospital during your first hours:

• Ask your nurse to write down the names of the doctors and nurses who are treating you.
• Try to get a transistor radio (listen to the news stations that broadcast the traffic, weather, and time).
• Ask the nurses to open the window shades (be aware of daytime and nighttime).
• Ask for paper and pens or pencils and a clipboard. Place a pillow under the clipboard to make writing more comfortable.
• Get your room TV turned on, but don't be surprised if the noise level and the daytime programs are not helpful for your new-patient feelings. The same game show you enjoyed at home may annoy you when you are in a hospital room.

Today, you need to learn to remain in your hospital bed. If you have bathroom privileges, try to make your trips in straight lines: bed to bathroom, bathroom to bed. If you can manage to stay in bed through your first hospital supper, the evening will pass quickly.

In these first hours, you may be receiving medication, orally or through an I.V. drip. Talk to your nurses about expected side effects, but don't try to tough it out if you feel uncomfortable. When you experience a side effect, it is an indication to the health-care team that the medication is doing something in your body. Talking to your nurse about how you are reacting to the medication provides information to your health-care team.

During these first few hours, you may also receive a visit from a clergyman of your faith. A nonmedical bedside visit will be a welcome relief. Clergy who perform duties in hospitals often have just the right words of comfort for you and your family at this time.

After the hospital supper, there is a visiting time, when the maternity ward seems a bit active. A special maternity snack is served in the evening.

The maternity snack came at 8:30 P.M. and I didn't feel like eating it. But my husband asked the nurse if he could have a snack, too. She and I realized that he hadn't eaten all day after I had been admitted. So he ate the sandwich, and she brought us some hot tea. Watching him eat, realizing how tired he was, I felt so sorry for us. There were so many changes we were going to have to make in our lives and he was going home to an empty apartment. For the rest of my hospital stay, and when I was on bedrest at home, we always had a maternity snack in the evening; it was a time when we ate our sandwiches and appreciated each other.

The maternity ward becomes very quiet by 10:00 P.M. Patients start to sleep, the evening shift closes out their work and waits for the night shift to come on duty. You may be concerned about how well you can sleep in a hospital. We can assure you that you will feel as though you had just driven six hundred miles and had checked into a motel room. Your exhaustion will overcome the strangeness of the room and bed and you will fall asleep.

If you are a parent, you've already handled the care of your children for the first emergency hours. Just make arrangements for the next day; you will be able to make better decisions tomorrow. And no matter how worried you feel, your voice on the telephone will greatly reassure your children. If you can, try to give them their own good-night phone call—you can make up a bedtime story or ask how the school day was and what your children are going to wear the next day.

Your First Full Day in the Hospital

When you woke up this morning, you were probably surprised that you actually did sleep. During the night, you heard voices outside your room, a nurse may have visited you to take your vital signs. Then early this morning your vital signs were taken again, and you might have gotten out of bed to be weighed. All this before 7:00 A.M.

This morning you may be prepared, "prepped," for a surgical procedure, or you may be scheduled for medical tests. Or none of the above. No matter what is planned for your day, you will spend a good part of it waiting.

Ask your nurse to tell you the mealtimes, when residents visit patients, visiting hours, and times for medical tests. When you list these activities, you'll see that a hospital day has certain active times and then hours when nothing happens. Now that you have a better idea of your free time you can do the following:

1. If you are currently working, and if you haven't read it already, read Chapter 15, "Your Job."
2. Use this list to check off what you want in your room:

___ 2–3 hangers (the hospital never seems to have enough).
___ Your current favorite low-heeled shoes—it's not necessary to wear slippers in a hospital. You can use nylon "peds" with your shoes.

___ A lightweight robe—you will need a robe when you leave your room. Hospitals are warm places and a lightweight cotton or polyester wrapper may be a better fabric than a cozy flannel or fleece robe.*

___ A coin purse, filled—the gift shop usually sends a cart around the hospital, filled with newspapers, magazines, and toiletries.

___ A bag of toiletries for yourself.

___ A Thermos bottle for making hot drinks without constantly calling nurses. As a rule, hospitals do not like patients to have their own food. Nurses may prefer to fill your Thermos with hot water and then supply you with tea bags, sugar, and instant coffee.

___ Your maternity bras. A friend can help you soak them in your sink and hang them up in your room bathroom.

___ Your address book and your local directories—when you are not looking up a phone number, the Yellow Pages is a flat surface to rest paper, books, even your food.

___ Lightweight hair dryer.

___ A craft project.

3. Talk to your nurse about visiting times for your children. Your nurse may advise continuing telephone calls until your medical condition is stabilized. There are hospital rules for the minimum age of visitors. Children can carry contagious illnesses that could make you sick or spread to the nursery. But don't be discouraged. Many hospitals have developed specific programs for young children and their hospitalized mothers. Often antepartum high-risk wards have special visiting rules for families that allow for young children to spend time with their mothers.

---

* *Note*: we did not include nightgowns in this list. The hospital will supply you with a fresh gown as often as you need one. You won't be making a fashion statement with the current designs, but these gowns make physical examinations very easy. The hospital laundry won't wash personal gowns. Here's a trick if your hospital gown is just not covering enough of you: wear two—one opens in the back, you wear the second like a short-sleeved wrap, opening in the front. It looks better than you might think.

4. Talk to each child's teachers. They should be aware that your child is dealing with a very stressful experience. The school counselor could provide support which is also helpful for you.

5. Call the admissions office if your roommate is a new mother. If you are in a maternity ward, we strongly urge you not to room with a new mother. She is up at all hours, has many visitors, and keeps her baby with her. You may find that you are answering the telephone, talking to grandparents, and responding to questions about your medical problems.

You have a right to rest in a room without this stress. You may need your doctor to initiate the room change and have the nursing staff help you. If your room currently has an empty second bed, request that this bed not be filled by a new mother.

Happily, many hospitals now have special wings or halls for high-risk expectant women. Your roommate may also be on bedrest. But even in this situation, your roommate may be having treatments or other difficulties that are stressful for you. Again, don't hesitate to request a change in your room.

I was staying in the hospital for some medical tests during my sixteenth week. Suddenly, I learned I was being moved to a room across the hallway. The expectant woman in that room was not staying on bedrest and one nurse had decided that I would have a good effect on her. I felt very badly for that other patient. But I told the nurses, in very strong words, that it was not my job to provide counseling to another patient, that I was a patient myself. I refused to move. A social worker saw the woman later that day.

The Next Few Days

It's rare to discharge a high-risk pregnant woman after one day of hospitalization. More likely, your minimum hospital stay will be about five days. During this time, your doctor can judge the success of a medical procedure and the medication you have been receiving. After a few days, the effect of remaining on bedrest in a specific position can be judged.

During these days, you will become more adjusted to the hospital routine. You'll begin to recognize the morning sounds of the night-shift nursing staff leaving and begin to joke with the nurses who wake you for vital signs. You'll enjoy being served meals and planning the next day's menus. Sleep will be easier and the daily activities will be increased.

You may be visited by a physical therapist. Certain pregnancy exercises may be continued throughout this period. The therapist will show you these and related exercises as well as devise a time schedule for your daily workout. You may also be visited by an occupational therapist, who will help you adjust to your side-lying position for your daily activities.

A hospital dietitian may visit and help you plan choices for menus that are compatible with your medical condition and the number of calories you should be consuming each day.

You may also receive a visit from a social worker who has valuable information concerning the social services available to pregnant women, and can help you talk about your feelings.

Work with your nurse to arrange appointment times that are compatible with your own daily schedule. For example, if you have settled into taking a short nap at 3:00 P.M., it would be best to have a health professional visit you after this nap when you are rested, or earlier in the day when you are not feeling sleepy.

Going Home

After a few days, your doctor will be able to judge whether you can continue in a medically stable condition at home or need the closer monitoring of the high-risk-pregnancy ward staff.

It's important to understand that your good efforts at maintaining your physical position and undergoing all the medical tests have *not* been for the goal of going home. Your doctor's decision to discharge you from the hospital is a judgment based on your medical condition today. If your medical condition changes, you may need to check into the hospital again. Rehospitalization is *not* a failure but simply another stage in your pregnancy that requires close monitoring by hospital staff.

> When I checked out of the hospital at sixteen weeks, I jokingly left my special scented hangers with the nursing staff. Just in case, I said. Well, at twenty-six weeks I was back again, and there, in my hospital room closet, were my hangers!

If your doctor recommends your discharge, talk seriously with him or her about a transition period of at least one day. Your home has to be ready for your return, completely set up for your bedrest. If this is the first time you will actually be managing bedrest by yourself, certain limitations that are part of hospitalization will no longer apply at home. Work with your nurse to complete the "Checklist: Hospital to Home" in Appendix 4.

Discharge Day

Once a date is set for your discharge from the hospital, concentrate on getting your home ready before you walk in the door. Now is a good time to reread other chapters in this book for setting up your home for bedrest. Family members and friends can use the lists in earlier chapters. You can make a diagram of your bedrest room. When family and friends have completed their work, they can snap a few instant photos of your redesigned room and bring them to the hospital for your approval.

The time that you can be discharged will vary based on your specific medical complication. Certain complications travel best in the morning, others in the evening. The person who is taking you to your home has to make adjustments in his or her workday. Your children have a schedule, too. Talk to your doctor and your nurse about all of these potential problems to determine the best time physically and emotionally for you to be released from the hospital.

The process of leaving the hospital can be very tiring for you.

Your belongings have to be packed, you have discharge discussions with your doctor, you have to get back into the wheelchair, go down to the hospital patient accounts office, settle your account, and then wait, still sitting up, for your transportation home. Minimize this stress by arranging for the patient accounts clerk to telephone you at your bedside or come up to the ward to complete your medical claim forms. Delay the wheelchair ride until your transportation is at the door, motor running. Handle the packing during a family member or friend's visit the night before your discharge.

Every high-risk pregnant woman enjoys the trip home. You get to feel the weather, hot summer air or gusts of winter wind. You see more sky, you see streets, and you hear traffic noises. Your driver may be tempted to give you a scenic tour or ask if you want to stop briefly for an errand. Try to resist any delays in getting home.

Put yourself in reverse gear and remember your first few hours of hospitalization: the rushing around, the confusion, and your exhaustion. That's what this first day home will be like. You are returning to a bedroom totally redesigned for bedrest. It may be difficult to reorient yourself the first evening.

The difference in this reorientation to home bedrest is that you are starting for the second time. All the skills you developed during your hospital bedrest make this first evening and the next few days easier. As you settle in, reread parts of this book, because certain ideas will now make more sense than they did when you read them in your hospital room.

20

*

Extended
Hospitalization

After several days, your doctor may determine that close monitoring by the hospital staff is necessary to enable your pregnancy to progress until the birth of your baby. You will probably remain in this hospital room, with the same schedule, until your final trip to the labor and delivery rooms.

If your doctor had told you this news the day you were admitted, you would have been much more upset than you are now. Still, it is depressing to know you'll be a hospital patient for a long time. But remind yourself that the medical procedures, the medication, and the prescribed bedrest positioning are allowing your baby to continue to grow inside of you.

You've made an adjustment to the hospital schedule, all the monitoring, even the food, and you're even beginning to get used to side-lying and/or elevating your hips in one position for long periods of time. You've mastered the mechanics of your hospital bed and feel a little burst of happiness when you change into a fresh hospital gown and it still has all its tie strings.

Welcome to the "cutting edge" of maternal-fetal medicine. As a patient, you will be managed by a highly skilled team of doctors, doctors-in-training (residents), and a full variety of nurses, all providing you with the most advanced medical treatments. But living, or rather, lying, on the cutting edge of medicine, can be painful.

First, your treatment is so different from other pregnancies that you can't share your hospital experience with friends who had more routine treatment. Their reaction to the news that you are receiving medication or being monitored may be confusion. They may ask you why you need so many tests and drugs. You begin to worry if all this medical monitoring is affecting you and your pregnancy. If you are spending your days in the high-risk antepartum ward, you may look forward to sharing experiences with other women undergoing the same treatment. But medical monitoring varies from patient to patient in this hospital ward, too. You and your roommate may have the same medical complications but be monitored and medicated differently.

Another particularly sharp point in the cutting edge of medicine is the constant adjustments in how your medical condition is managed. Every morning, you and several residents exchange questions and answers about your medical condition. One morning, you hear that the delivery date will be in several weeks. Later that morning a nurse comments that you'll probably deliver your baby in ten days. The residents thought you'd need a Cesarean section. Your personal doctor (attending physician) tells you that you might be able to deliver vaginally. Every time a staff member mentions a birth date or a change in treatment, you have to change your plans and ready yourself. After a few days, you may be tempted to march your entire high-risk medical team into your room's bathroom, lock the door, and not let them out until they've made up their minds.

Actually, gathering your medical team at your bedside and telling them all at once how you feel is not a bad idea. You know that the strategy of managing your pregnancy is being constantly adjusted as your medical condition stabilizes or changes. You have to decide for yourself whether you want to participate in the process of managing your pregnancy or whether you want bedside conversations limited to what is absolutely certain. You decide what is best for you and make sure the medical staff fully understands what you want said or discussed at your bedside.

The cutting edge also has some dull spots. You are living in a room in a corridor that never changes. The temperature stays about the same (warm!), the nurses and hospital staff dress in either whites or surgical scrubs, and the furniture is exactly the same in each room. There are no weekends in a hospital; the routine is the same seven days a week. The sameness of hospital scenery and routine can make you feel tired and depressed. Every patient who is hospitalized for longer than a few days, for any medical problem, experiences this exhaustion and sadness. Periods of hospital depression are a normal part of the week.

You can overcome hospital depression with the same tools and tricks described in the other chapters of this book. Start with Chapter 8, "Planning Your Days," to develop your own weekly schedule. Use Chapter 6, "Setting Up Your Room," for ways to personalize your hospital room. For example, arrange to have a series of travel posters pasted on a wall at a height you can see easily. Be sure to have those pictures changed once a week. You could trade pictures with other hospitalized women—a sort of traveling art exhibit.

Your occupational therapist may suggest ways to occupy the long hours between meals and medical tests. Read Chapter 17, "Expanding Your Horizons," to identify short-term and long-term projects you would like to try. Also, hospitals have video cassette players for educational films. Ask if you can borrow the machine for a few hours and watch a movie.

You will still need to solve many of the tough problems of child care, extended leave from your job, medical costs, and rearrangement of your family budget that are covered in other chapters. Since you will be using the telephone all day, you may want to attach some accessories to the handset, or use a more convenient phone set, as described in Chapter 5, "Basic Equipment." Be sure to discuss with the hospital engineer the changes you want to make.

Encourage weekly visiting times for your friends. Your friends can join you in watching a movie or can bring a board game. For these scheduled visits, you may feel happier wearing pregnancy pants and a loose top. Ask for permission to change into street clothes.

Being in a hospital makes you accessible to unexpected visitors, and during visiting hours, you may find a surprise guest. These visitors mean well and in the midst of their own schedule have finally found a day to get to the hospital and bring you some flowers and cheer. They assume, as most hospital visitors do, that you are waiting all day for visiting hours and are prepared to receive them. Most of the time you're not. It's amazing how quickly a visiting coworker will forget about your hospital bed and gossip about an office issue. Chapter 26, "Your Friends," describes how to minimize sick calls.

If a visitor pops in, sits down for a chat, and you feel trapped, try to send a special signal to your nurse. Work out a code of words so that when your nurse hears your message of help, she can respond and gently remove your visitor.

Sometimes a period of depression sets in that doesn't respond to your plan of the day. In this instance, scrap all your plans, and declare a silly day. Read joke books. Ask to rent a truly funny film. Demand that every member of your medical team attempt to tell you a funny joke. Ask your dietitian to make a silly meal tray. Laughter can take the dull ache out of a depressed day.

If intensive work at laughter is not lightening your mood, you may want to identify the source of your depression and, perhaps, read the next chapter. There are many reasons for blue days in a pregnancy. You may need to talk to a social worker during this time who can help you sort out your feelings.

Your Family

Your family is beginning to adjust to your hospitalization. The news that you are going to stay for a while is probably less upsetting to your family than was your initial admission to the hospital. They've started to get used to your early-morning and good-night phone calls. Your children may have visited you and seen that their mother still looks the same and has nurses helping her.

In fact, your family and friends are going to go on with their lives, feeling confident and relaxed knowing you're being cared for by professional hospital staff. Children are going to learn about their father's cooking and cleaning skills; they may start to do some chores themselves. Your mother or his mother may move in for a while and help the way a grandmother can. Or your children may go on an extended visit to their grandparents, even attend another school for a while, perhaps the school you attended.

Their ability to handle this difficult period well does not mean your family does not need you. It means you've been a good parent who has given her children the necessary strength to cope with this situation.

The Evanston Hospital, a regional perinatal center in Illinois, has developed an Infant Care Program providing a special set of activities for bedrest mothers who have extended hospitalizations. For some families, the staff recommends that a mother tape-record herself reading a children's story or relating some personal news. This cassette tape is then given to her child (or children) who can play it back on a children's cassette player. Often this child feels that he has lost the ability to make his mother respond directly to his needs when she is far away in a hospital bed. With the cassette tape, the child can start and stop his mother, gaining back some ability to interact with her. The Evanston Hospital staff also works directly with children, preparing them for the birth of a premature sibling with special tours of the neonatal wing and talks with child development professionals.

If you have been displaying refrigerator schoolwork and art, you can duplicate your refrigerator in your room. A hospital staff member or friend can use colored tape to paste an outline of a refrigerator on one wall. Your children's artwork remains on the "refrigerator." Be sure to rotate the work once a week to keep yourself up to date. What a nice surprise for your children to see their current work in your room.

If your children can't visit, arrange to have some pictures taken of yourself and developed every few days. That way your children can see your pregnancy develop. The pictures can be of the newest refrigerator display, your favorite breakfast tray, a project you are making for them; even the hospital staff can pose for pictures.

Start a garden. Ask a friend to plant radish seeds or lima beans or flower seeds in a flat bed that fits onto the window ledge. Seedlings grow at a rate you can watch, and they can travel home with you. It's a great project for you to do with your children or to share in pictures.

Couples

This is also a time of great stress for fathers and mothers. You may want to read the chapters in the next section, "Taking Stock of All the Changes," about couples, emotions, and family stories. Fathers have unlimited visiting privileges, which can help restore some intimacy to the relationship. Many bedresters have received permission to have fathers spend the night. The doorknob can be hung with a DO NOT DISTURB sign.

> As the days passed, he looked more and more exhausted. I got permission for him to spend the night with me. He cheerfully ate the special guest supper, finished an extra maternity snack, and within moments of settling into bed, was sound asleep. Snuggled against my special human bolster, I slept well for the first time.

Discharge from the Hospital

Some pregnant bedresters may spend several weeks in the hospital followed by several weeks at home on bedrest. Most of the time, long-term hospitalization continues until childbirth or pregnancy loss. Afterward, you will quickly be back on your feet again. Many hospitals reassign a new mother from an antepartum high-risk wing to the maternity ward after her child is born. After several weeks spent among other bedresters, the maternity ward feels like a different hospital. Pregnancy bedresters, whether they were on bedrest at home or in a hospital, experience common postpartum feelings described in chapters 28, "The First Days of Motherhood," and 29, "It's All Over—or Is It?"

When you are finally back on your feet again, you will begin making plans for going home. Just like the bedresters who traveled home after a short hospital stay, you will experience an exhilarating ride home, almost overwhelmed by the variety of colors and street scenes you have missed.

It is important for you to recognize that feeling disoriented for a few days is a normal part of the adjustment to home life after a long period of hospitalization. The members of your medical team, especially your physical therapist, can help you develop a routine of activities that will build your strength as you resume your lifestyle.

*

TAKING STOCK OF
ALL THE CHANGES

*

21

*

Your Emotions

High-risk pregnancy is a time of intense emotions coupled with unpredictable change. Aside from the enormous stress of staying in bed, you have to find a way to tolerate all of the strong feelings that you have about your baby and yourself.

The minute your pregnancy is labeled high-risk, you may feel a strong sense of loss. You may no longer imagine yourself leading the active pregnant life you had hoped to lead. Your blissful pregnancy fantasies may be quickly replaced with visions of spending your days in bed. You can find it hard to recapture the image of yourself glowing with joy as you blossom through the months of gestation.

Your mental picture of a healthy, full-term baby might begin to fade. You can still hope for that child, but you can also see yourself with a tiny preemie. Almost anyone who experiences such a blow to her fantasies will react much like someone who is grieving. At first there is shock. You remember little of what was said to you. You may doubt the diagnosis or think the recommended treatment is too extreme—especially if you feel physically normal. You are confused and numb.

Anticipating Bedrest

Some of you will be told that bedrest is probable in a later stage of your pregnancy. If you are carrying more than one baby, had a previous premature birth, a history of premature labor, or known cervical problems, your doctor may recommend that you begin bedrest when you reach a certain number of weeks in pregnancy and your uterus begins to get heavy. This advance warning gives you some time to prepare your mind and organize your life around the coming change. Some women, like the mother quoted below, develop their own special ways of coping with anticipation.

I was the queen of magical thinking before my planned bedrest began at twenty-nine weeks. Trying to deny my fears and the amount of risk involved, I imagined that I was utterly safe until the exact day on which I was to go to bed. Somehow, I would make an overnight transformation from a normal pregnancy to one that required me to lie down at all times.

On my last day I shopped like a maniac for baggy sundresses, sweat suits, books, craft projects—anything to avoid going home. I arrived home with heavy shopping bags and a tired body. Did this stop me from having a farewell restaurant dinner? No! As we strolled around after dinner enjoying the last of the summer breezes that I would feel for some time, I became aware of my uterus begging me to take things seriously. Feeling contractions, I could no longer continue my escape and reluctantly went home to bed.

The First Day

Once you begin bedrest, you may experience the First Day Blues, the overwhelmed feelings that most women have on their first day of bedrest whether they went to bed suddenly or had months to prepare. The First Day Blues are just that; usually they are limited to the first day or two of bedrest. Your first feelings of depression will pass and you will discover inner strength and courage, if not on your first or second morning, perhaps on your third day. Meanwhile, be patient and kind to yourself as you begin to develop a routine for passing the time.

The Next Few Days

Congratulations, you have made it through your first day in bed! This may seem like small potatoes compared to all the days you will need to be there, but believe us when we say that you should celebrate your accomplishment. Few days are as difficult as that first one—the day you realized how often you would have to ask for help, how much you did on foot that must now be covered by others, and how small your bedroom really is.

In these next days, you will begin to find the energy to make some practical plans and think about how you will entertain yourself. These positive moments will be mixed with fear for your baby and times when you are too upset or distracted to focus on getting things done. You may still have periods when you cannot admit to yourself how serious your problems are.

As in any experience of loss or grief, you can find yourself becoming angry, searching for good reasons for the complications, looking for someone to blame, and perhaps feeling guilty for something you did that might have caused your trouble. This is one of the times that bedresters often feel depressed. It can be hard to get through these feelings, especially if you don't feel free to talk about them. Since you are so dependent on your caregivers, it can be uncomfortable to share strong, negative feelings with them. Usually it helps to find a friend who can listen. At this point, some women turn to bedrest support groups and some to professional counselors.

> I was seeing a therapist during my pregnancy and I found his support to be vital for me in handling all of my fears, frustration, hopes, and anger. This was one place where I could say anything—one person who did not feed me, take care of my child, sleep with me, do my laundry, examine my

body, or give me good and bad news about my baby. Early in my bedrest, I continued to go for my appointments, since his office was a few blocks from my obstetrician—attention for my mind and body in one outing! I would lie down on a couch during my sessions and feel foolish about it since I normally sat in a chair. I never told my obstetrician that I was going because I was worried that he would think I was really unstable if I needed therapy. In hindsight, I doubt that he would have been so judgmental.

It is so easy at this stage to assume that women in normal pregnancies are breezing along, cheerfully leading their lives as though their growing bellies make no difference in their daily routines or outlook. Nothing could be further from the truth! Pregnancy itself is a time of enormous emotional change, full of turmoil, confusion, and ambivalence along with the expected joys. You are now actually coping with three major changes: pregnancy, medical risk, and bedrest. Any one of these could be difficult all by itself!

As Your Bedrest Continues

Once the first few days have passed, you will find yourself getting into your own daily patterns and schedules. The initial shock of diagnosis is over, but the emotional adjustment continues. In spite of your many good days now, there can be a subtle undercurrent of grief over the loss of a normal pregnancy and sadness as you anticipate possible harm to yourself or your child.

Another stage in coping with these painful feelings is the onset of bargaining. You may beg your doctor to say that it is safe to go to the movies or to take a walk. This bargaining comes out of some magical belief that if the doctor says it's okay, it guarantees the extra activity is risk-free. How wonderful it would be if someone could really know precisely what behavior is safe! You might make bargains with God: "I'll never argue with anyone again and always do volunteer work if you let this baby make it." You can get superstitious ideas that "all will go well if I don't wear my old maternity clothes. . . . If I don't buy anything for the new baby, I won't feel so sad if I never bring him home." Bargaining begins to fade eventually, usually when you feel ready to know more of the facts about your pregnancy.

Three Stress Factors

Pregnancy

Normal pregnancy can be a highly emotional state for the expectant mother. If this is your first pregnancy, you have a short nine months in which to transform yourself from the person you have been all of your life to that unknown role called "mother." Sometimes it feels as if the baby will be ready before you are! There are days when you feel confident about your new job and days when you're sure that you are not cut out to be a mom. Most expectant mothers have their secret moments when they are convinced that the pregnancy was a big mistake. You wonder how your relationship with your partner will change when the baby arrives, how big your body will get, and how long it will take to look normal again (if ever). You worry about your sex appeal and wonder if all hope is gone for that backpacking adventure in Tibet.

The whole world treats you differently. Strangers touch your belly and give unsolicited advice. Professional colleagues act a little awkward around you. Some are self-conscious about looking at you; some behave as though your brain has turned to mush. They tone down their language since you're a mother now and presumably will be offended by swearing, flirting, or dirty jokes. You feel tempted to shout, "Hey, everybody, it's still me!"

If all this doesn't get to you, your hormones will make you moody without any help from the outside world. A woman who is usually rational and moderate in her approach to daily life may be shocked to find herself bursting into tears during a sentimental television commercial, or raging at her husband over a minor disagreement.

Medical Risk

When you learn that your baby's healthy arrival is in doubt, your coping skills are severely challenged. Suddenly you have an un-answered question that will not be resolved for months: will this baby be okay? You can ignore the question for brief periods of time, but it is never far from your thoughts. It creates an unspoken undercurrent of anxiety. Faced with a risky pregnancy, you may feel uncertain about whether or not to make plans for the baby. You may try not to care too much in hopes that you will feel less pain if things go poorly. When these feelings aren't consciously on your mind, they may go underground and lead to a vague sense of tension, irritability, or loss. You don't feel good, but you're not sure why.

You may become openly tearful, angry, depressed, or afraid as you try to go about your life, all the time knowing that something bad could happen. Some mothers say that they feel like their body is a time bomb or a volcano waiting to erupt.

Bedrest

Bedrest causes its own stress and strain. It requires coping on a day-to-day basis with physical limitations, changes in relationships, a restructuring of time, and the sense of being trapped, without time off for good behavior. Even people who are not pregnant but who are on prescribed bedrest for minor conditions have extraordi-nary difficulty coping with it.

Perhaps the worst aspect of bedrest is the monotony. In a normal day, you would be unable to count the thousands of sights, sounds, aromas, tastes, and textures that reach your senses and enter your mind. So much of this stimulation is unconsciously received. You can remember the taste of that wonderful soup at lunch and the sound of singing as you walked past a church, but you have no idea of the number of instant pleasures that your brain noted today while you were concentrating on other things. There was the smooth touch of your leather handbag, the warm hug of your coat against the crisp breeze, the bird's song, the flash of brilliant blue as the clouds cleared for a moment, the fragrance of fresh bread near the bakery, the rhythmic slap of your feet on the sidewalk, the burst of peppermint from a stick of gum.

When you are in bed, there are few treats for your senses, and your mind reacts accordingly. You may find yourself daydreaming more, seeming to hear more acutely or being less able to pay attention to voices in the distance, feeling tingling sensations in your legs as if they had fallen asleep, losing your sense of time or season. These are common responses to lack of stimulation.

Numerous bedresters have talked about being in a time warp. They feel like their bedrest was lost time, so it makes no sense that the seasons have continued to change, the holidays arrive and end, the normal flow of life continues. Some women tell us that they continued to feel a few months behind the calendar long after they gave birth. With all these changes, is it any wonder that bedrest is tough?

Emotional Coping from This Point On

Over time, you will develop your own personal style of coping with the sometimes dramatic, sometimes boring days of your bedrest pregnancy. You will be amazed to catch yourself so completely distracted that you forgot about your situation. Maybe it will be in the middle of a belly laugh over a funny book or movie, maybe in an intense conversation with a friend about *her* life. Naturally, there will be good days and bad days—days when you feel angry or scared or sad, days when you think you can't stand another moment in bed. You will learn to accept these ups and downs as normal. You will learn to say to yourself, "Today I'll do nothing and probably cry a lot. That's okay; tomorrow I'll feel better." You will find yourself gaining new strength, a sense of acceptance and a willingness to do what is necessary for your baby. In order to be able to handle the occasional bad times, it will help you to know some of the common reasons for difficulty.

Knowing Why You Are Upset Helps

When you experience a bad day or the onset of the blues, try to sort out the source of your feelings. Sometimes you can take comfort in knowing that you are having the mood swings that all pregnant women have. Hormone changes and fatigue could be to blame. At other times, your bedrest restrictions or your medical concerns could be the reason for your mood.

If you are having crying bouts every few days, try keeping a short daily diary to see if you can find any pattern to the crying spells. Do they come at a certain time of the day? Do they follow contact with a specific person? Are there predictable events or feelings that occur before the crying begins? Identifying a pattern or a cause will help you to interrupt the cycle and to weather the occasional stormy day knowing that it will pass, as storms always do.

Some of the reasons for having a good day are obvious: having a happy visit to the doctor's office, reaching a time when your baby could be born safely, getting a test result that indicates your pregnancy is progressing well, receiving a supportive phone call, hearing your partner say, "I love you." Many reasons for feeling bad are obvious, too: further restrictions in your routine, unexpected hospitalization, medication side effects, cranky children, an exhausted spouse. Sometimes, however, knowing why you are feeling happy or blue is not so easy.

One morning, I was bored from the minute I woke up. I cried about everything. I told Ray I was bored, so he started giving me a huge list of ideas. They all sounded boring to me and I yelled at him to leave me alone. My friends called and everybody had something they thought I should try. I didn't think any of them really understood what it was like to lie here so long. Each time I tried to do one of my craft projects, I couldn't concentrate. Then I saw this darling little baby on a commercial and the floodgates opened. I sobbed for so long. I thought I was bored all day, but really I was scared. I was worrying without even knowing it because I had to go have this special test done the next day. When I realized what the problem was, I called my doctor's office and asked them a million questions. That helped. When Ray came home, I told him how scared I was and he said he was, too.

Once this mother identified worry rather than boredom as the source of her irritation, she was able to do things to help herself.

Sometimes the Trouble Is an Anniversary

Another very common experience for women who have had previous pregnancies is the anniversary reaction. You have significant dates in your life, such as birthdays, wedding anniversaries, the day you bought a house, the day your grandmother died. Happy or sad, these are days that come each year and remind you of something important. The date stands out on your calendar because you have strong feelings about the event that took place.

When you reach the point at which something went wrong in your previous pregnancy, you could become upset even though your current pregnancy is not in immediate danger. Some of these anniversary dates are calendar days: "My premature labor started on May 23." If you are pregnant again on May 23, that may be an anxious day.

Some anniversaries are remembered as stages of pregnancy: "I was hospitalized at twenty-six weeks." Twenty-six weeks into the next pregnancy, you might find yourself remembering the hospital, or becoming inexplicably blue. However you count these days, they tend to be milestones in the next pregnancy. Your strong feelings as you approach one of these significant times are a normal reaction to a difficult experience. Getting past a milestone can be a great relief.

When I was about seventeen weeks pregnant, I got so anxious. I began to have this terrible feeling that the baby would die. I cried a lot and Joe and I argued about anything and everything. He was a mess, too. A few weeks later, I realized that I felt good again. Joe said, "Well, we made it longer this time," and suddenly I knew what was going on. Last time, I miscarried at eighteen weeks and we both must have been just waiting for it to happen again. Somehow passing eighteen weeks made us feel a whole lot more confident about this baby.

I Need a Vacation!

Being in the same situation day after day will sometimes overwhelm you. You might think, "If only I could get away from my room and my bed for just one afternoon, I would be fine." You would simply like to have some time out. All pregnant women have an occasional burning desire to put their bellies in storage for a day. When this happens, they are able to cheer themselves by visiting a museum, hiding in a movie theater, strolling through a mall, or going for a drive—all options that you don't have.

This is the moment when temptation rears its ugly head. You wonder if a small outing would really be so bad. If you and your doctor think that some outings are not harmful, this is the time to go. If you know that it is probably too risky to be active, do anything that you can to keep your promise to yourself to stay in bed. The joy of escape can too quickly be replaced by fear and guilt if your condition worsens. Mothers are very talented at blaming themselves when things go wrong (no matter why there was a problem), so don't add any fuel to the fire.

When the urge to escape really builds, you *can* leave the room. This is the time to have someone build a second nest in your home for a change of scenery. Once your plans are carried out, you can spend parts of your day in different places in the house or apartment. Make an agreement with yourself that you will only change nests when you are up anyway for a trip to the bathroom. You can carry the telephone along with you as you move. Some bedresters have actually changed houses by spending the weeks between doctor visits with a relative and returning home after the next appointment. This gives their partner a small break from routine and a time to relax, knowing that the mother is in good hands.

Who Owns This Body?

One of the hardest challenges you will face during bedrest is that of maintaining your self-esteem and creating a positive self-image. Medical diagnoses of "incompetent cervix" or "irritable uterus" may make you feel personally incompetent or emotionally irritable. Perhaps you have always enjoyed good health and this is the first time you have been told there is something wrong with your body. Or you may have ongoing medical problems and now one of these problems is not only worsening, but is affecting the life of your baby, as well. You can no longer take the functioning of your body for granted. Whether your medical problem is dangerous for you or not, you can feel afraid for yourself during this time.

Indeed, the things you always assumed that you could control now seem to be out of your hands. You may be accustomed to planning your life in great detail, including getting pregnant at a time of year that was convenient for you. Suddenly it feels like doctors and fate are calling the shots. This could be one of the first times in your life that you haven't been successful at deciding things for yourself and, if you like to have a sense of control, it can be a blow to your self-esteem to be transformed into someone who needs to ask so much of others.

One woman managed to keep her sense of self with the help of a caring nurse:

> One nurse made it easy because she saw me as a real person. She always talked to me and she explained everything in detail. I looked forward to seeing her face. I don't know how I would have made it so long without her.

Sometimes in dealing with your medical problems and your dependence on others, you may begin to think of yourself as a weak, sick, or passive person. How long can anyone lie in bed and not feel sick or disabled? Concentrate on viewing yourself as an assertive woman who is managing to cope with a difficult situation. You may need help to accomplish many daily tasks, but you can be active in arranging for that help. There are also things that you can still do by yourself and on which you can focus your attention. Some women say that it helps their spirits to do something "public" in addition to protecting their pregnancy. They may volunteer to help a charity or school by making phone calls or stuffing envelopes. Other women find that managing their own lives is all they want to tackle at this complicated time. Think of yourself as a well person who temporarily needs to be in bed. If you take medication and do feel ill, this, too, is usually a temporary situation; the medication and ill feeling will most likely disappear after the pregnancy.

The women who cope best with a high-risk pregnancy are those who show their feelings, actively seek help, and make a real effort to see themselves as competent participants in the treatment team. You may feel out of control and there are certainly things that you cannot change, but you are the one who decides who will be on your medical team and what recommendations you will accept.

Many of our suggestions about clothing and personal grooming will help promote a positive attitude. Think of yourself as a special kind of athlete who needs to eat carefully, rest properly, and prepare mentally and physically for a scheduled athletic event—your baby's birth. The medical team coaches you, your family and friends cheer you, but you are the one who runs the race.

I Would Like a Good Cry Now. . . .

So what do you do if you have identified the reason for the bad feelings, communicated with others about them, sought information, tried solutions—and nothing helps? This is the time for a good cry. Give in, beat the pillow, throw a few items at the walls, and get that tension out of your system. We recommend throwing a light object such as a Nerf ball, since it will give your arm muscles some exercise and won't damage walls or shatter. It may seem absurd to picture yourself throwing sponge balls and sobbing, but nature gave you the ability to cry for sound reasons. A good cry relieves stress and allows you to gather your coping skills once again.

If you are at risk for premature labor, you may find that the contractions increase with energetic crying. Talk to your doctor about this. It is impossible to tell you to hold back your tears, but try to release your frustration slowly, like letting the air out of a balloon.

How Your Family Reacts to Your Emotional Changes

As a wife, mother, daughter, and sister, you are an integral part of a family. Changes in your life affect those around you. There will be times when family members seem to be right in rhythm with you, meeting your needs graciously and competently.

My mother came to visit while I was in bed. Her presence and help with my daughter were such a comfort. I think I will always remember her massaging my feet while we talked. It was such a simple, soothing gesture that spoke to my weary heart as much as to my aching body.

Then there are those times when everybody has a crisis of his or her own and nobody can help. For most women in high-risk pregnancy, life is an uneven combination of the two.

In the next chapters, you will read about the ways in which family members react to your special pregnancy. They will often look to you for clues as to how to act and feel. When you feel confident and assertive, they will probably feel secure and treat you as someone who knows what she's doing. When you are in despair, some relatives will support you, some will avoid you, and some will be afraid. There will be days when you can shore up others emotionally and days when all you can do is take care of yourself.

It is in relation to their families that many women struggle with guilt during bedrest. You may worry about the burden that this situation places on other children and your partner. Feeling guilty implies that the problem is all your fault and somehow under your control. Wouldn't you be back on your feet if you could make the trouble go away? Surely you didn't choose this! It can be scary to realize that you don't have control over your complication, but accepting this truth can ease your guilt.

Just as individual women learn to cope with bedrest in stages, families go through the adjustment process, too. A whole family may be in shock, deny the risk, be angry, search for answers, blame, bargain, or accept. Their progress with coping will have its ups and downs. In some families, one person is full of denial while others accept the diagnosis and are ready to go to great lengths to accommodate the pregnancy. When individual family members are in different stages of coping, it is important to work together to come up with an acceptable plan of action.

Your Emotional Relationship with Doctors and Nurses

Many of the most emotional moments take place in the presence of doctors and nurses. They have the difficult task of telling women that their pregnancies are high-risk, recommending treatment options, and delivering the results of countless examinations and tests. Some health professionals are skilled in easing their patients through the first emotional minutes of receiving bad news. Others, though skilled in the diagnosis and management of a complicated pregnancy, find the emotional reactions of their patients painful and upsetting.

As a result of normal fears and anxiety, high-risk patients often react to bad news like lightning looking for the nearest place to strike. Medical people become an easy target because they deliver the bad news, perform the painful procedures, advise restricting your activities, and see you at your most vulnerable. You are quite literally naked with them. Because of your vulnerability, you can be extremely sensitive to the things these significant people say and the way they treat you. When they seem insensitive, your hurt and anger can be enormous.

Doctors and nurses are people, too. They have good days when things go well and bad days which leave them impatient or short-tempered. Since high-risk obstetricians work with so many difficult pregnancies, they often face disappointment. Sometimes a doctor or nurse simply doesn't have the patience to calm you when you are most upset.

One day during an examination, I asked at least a dozen times if my baby's head had truly grown to the size that meant it might survive if born. My doctor suddenly got very angry and told me there were plenty of taxi drivers who could deliver babies, too! I just lay on the table and cried. I learned later that he was treating an extremely critical pregnancy in another room. I also realized I was terribly tired of my complication. We had simply fought briefly.

When there are misunderstandings between you and the professionals who care for you, try to take a deep breath and a moment to think. In the great majority of cases, all of you have the same goal—the delivery of a healthy baby. No patient, doctor, or nurse should be treated rudely in the process, but some clashes are inevitable when so much is at stake. Try to let them know how you feel when they upset you and be willing to apologize when you are out of line.

The personal styles of patient and care provider may be comfortably complementary or quite different. It is easy for a take-charge doctor to work with a woman who wants a decisive physician who can reassure her. A woman who feels best when she knows all the facts fits more easily with a doctor who likes to educate and encourage patients to take an active role in decision making. It would be wonderful if all patients and care providers could be matched for personal style, but that just isn't realistic. For a high-risk pregnancy, appropriate medical skills are top priority.

Doctors and nurses are used to working with many different kinds of people and can usually adapt their style to fit a patient's needs. You can help to make this happen by being clear about your preferences. You can say, "All of that medical terminology scares me. I really need encouragement and reassurance." Or, "Please don't tell me everything will be okay. I would feel best if you gave me specific details about my condition." Or, "I can see that you worry when I am upset, but I really need to cry right now." Most doctors and nurses will be grateful for the information.

Taking a Positive Approach

When you need some good news, think about these facts:

- Obstetrical care is the best it has ever been and gets better every day.
- Survival rates for premature babies are at an all-time high, with each year bringing incredible advances.
- A bedrest pregnancy is a temporary situation. Most complications stop or greatly diminish immediately after childbirth.
- You are quickly learning skills that will serve you for your whole life—planning ahead, learning to ask for help, talking on the telephone and getting what you want.
- As a new mother, you'll have a head start. You'll know how to organize, live simply, grab a nap, and adapt to change.
- You are learning to be patient. This is going to make you a great mother.
- In just a few months or less, you are going to get up and get going.

You Are Doing a Great Job

It is important to remind yourself as often as you need to that each day you stay in bed is a real accomplishment toward your goal of having a healthy baby. The fact that you were in a bad mood one day, cried, threw a beanbag at a wall, felt sorry for yourself, and yelled at a family member can never detract from what is most important: you stayed in bed. If you only watch soap operas and game shows, read matchbook covers, and eat at regular intervals during the day, you can state with pride that you worked successfully at staying in bed. Well-meaning friends may suggest that you try to accomplish something. They might suggest that you earn a Ph.D. or teach yourself Arabic. These are fine goals if they interest you and help you, but staying in bed is a tremendous achievement—the most important one!

22

＊

Fathers' Voices

One day I threw a lemon meringue pie at the wall . . . part of it was because we have a two-story house and I would go back and forth fifteen times to do different things—up and down the stairs. And then one day, Elizabeth said, "Oh, you forgot the salt." And that was it! That's all it took—pie against the floor and the wall!

Next to you, the person who experiences the most changes during bedrest is the baby's father. He takes on enormous emotional burdens and physical tasks, yet he is seldom given an opportunity to talk about his reactions to the situation. Too often when your friends see him in the grocery store or driving the children to school, they ask him how *you* are and not how *he* is. Since men tend to count on their spouses for emotional support, they are often inexperienced at telling their personal worries to someone else. Many men feel very isolated in the midst of the whirlwind of high-risk pregnancy. Lots of people are around, but they all seem to focus on the mother.

It's easier to say to a woman who's confined, "Look, there's a support group," because that means something to a lot of women. You could have said that to me and I would have been very reticent to call anybody on the telephone.

Getting the News

Some fathers know in advance that the pregnancy is high-risk. Some experience the same shock and disbelief that many mothers encounter when hearing an unexpected diagnosis.

> I came home to an empty house. I had no idea where she was—actually, what happened was that my dad called and told me she was in the hospital, and they had Julie, our daughter, and I should go down there. My father said, "But, don't have a wreck getting there, it's not that bad—there's something wrong." When I hung up, Jan called me and said she was at the hospital and everything was okay, but I needed to come see her. . . . We had to talk and everything.
>
> *
>
> The doctor told us all the great news—no sex, no going up and down stairs, no standing to cook dinner, no just about anything—essentially, you can get up and go to the bathroom, and that's about it. I couldn't believe it—to start with, we already had a three-year-old.
>
> *
>
> We had been working with our doctor for about a year before the pregnancy. Sonia had had some surgery to remove a fibroid. We were geared and prepared for trouble and, in a sense, that made it easier. We knew what we were getting into.

Working with the Doctor

Being involved with medical professionals can bring out all sorts of intense feelings for fathers. Most are grateful to have an expert on the case. However, the knowledge and decision-making power of doctors can make some fathers feel even more out of control and powerless in an overwhelming situation.

I think the fact that he included both of us was very important; otherwise it would have been very easy for me to feel excluded. It helped a lot that there was somebody who she could lean on, somebody who was outside of the couple . . . who would be the source of emotional strength as well as professional advice. We had a very warm relationship— one that I value a great deal. I came to admire him enormously—a man of tremendous emotional strength and courage. I think it was important that she was getting this kind of support, not only from her husband, but from her physician as well.

*

I'm not real fond of doctors in general. This guy is not my favorite person. I didn't feel it was my role to tell Elizabeth that she should change doctors. It seemed to me that it was quite unreasonable to say she should be confined to bed and then insist that she come into the office. He didn't know how to deal with a professional woman who was very sophisticated in terms of medical issues.

*

The doctor was totally honest with us—that's one of the things I appreciated the most. A reasonably intelligent couple needs the honesty and forthrightness of a physician in order to have a good working relationship.

*

I needed to trust him. I felt, if nothing else, I needed to trust the man and he made it easy—his style and credentials. I hoped she'd find comfort in his counseling. I was relieved that I wasn't the sole source of support in this period of anxiety.

Paying the Bills

Just as large medical bills and fees for help stretch the family budget, income may be reduced by the mother's leaving work or the father's being less able to spend time and energy on his job.

> Though she was entitled to her accumulated sick leave and annual leave, we were basically down from two incomes to one, at a time when I wasn't making a really good salary, and so we were in more than a bit of a crunch. I've always done some free-lancing work and I tried to do as much of that as I could. It was a difficult year.
>
> *
>
> We went into debt a lot. We were fortunate that my parents were able to lend us money and I still owe them the money. It was one of those kinds of things where we just did it and we knew we had to do it and we're still in debt. It was something that came up frequently—we couldn't do something . . . because we didn't have any money. . . . Or we'd get to the end of the month and we didn't have the cash to pay the bills and had to put them off. That could lead to some friction because both of us would feel bad about that situation, but also there was no escape from it.

Effect on Work Life

In a family crisis, it becomes difficult to concentrate on work. Many fathers are at a life stage where they are working especially hard to establish themselves. Not all employers are understanding about the need for more time at home.

> [Early in the pregnancy]: I was very fortunate in that I can pretty much run my own schedule—that helped enormously. I had colleagues who were extraordinarily understanding and really didn't push me or pressure me very much. I managed to do everything I needed to do because I was very, very well organized . . . I had lots of lists.
>
> [Later in the same pregnancy]: It was all very anxiety producing and I figured it affected every aspect of our lives and certainly my own professional life. I think it was a time

when I had a great deal of difficulty concentrating on my work. I was always distracted by thoughts of this very tense emotional problem we had.

*

The year that Michelle was born, I went to a meeting and I told the secretary if anything happened, if Sonia needed me for any reason, to come over and get me. Well, at some point, she showed up in the room and I saw her walk through the door and she said to me, "No, it's for somebody else!" Apparently, I had turned, in a second, absolutely ashen white—I looked like I was about to drop dead.

Managing the Household

In the midst of this family emergency, the father is called upon to add new, unfamiliar duties to his already stressful day.

The burden was surprising, and I quickly realized that we were going to have to cooperate and communicate better than ever before. Fortunately, we decided to get some extra help. We had to borrow money to do it, but it was worth it. Between the three of us, regular household tasks were accomplished, but not without a significant change in our lifestyle.

*

I ended up doing all the grocery shopping and picking up things that were necessary around the house besides groceries—you know, stuff that men just don't normally have to do. Normally, you can look in the linen closet and you have shaving cream, razor blades in there. . . . It didn't take long for all that stuff to run out, so then I had to start doing all the surveying of the things that were necessary for the next week, or the next couple of weeks, and make lists, take care of those responsibilities.

*

I would get up in the morning and make her breakfast and bring it in to her in bed. We hired a young student to prepare lunch. Sonia was on a carefully regulated diet and so I would do the shopping very carefully. I would get cuts of veal, chicken, things that I knew she could have. They had to be served in fairly exact measurements, so I got measuring cups and scales and devices to use so that I would get the proportions correct.

*

Cooking—actually, it was a release for me. During the fifteen weeks that Elizabeth was confined, if you had asked me what the high points of those fifteen weeks were, it would be cooking. I cooked an entire Thanksgiving dinner from scratch, which I've never done before and I'll probably never do again. That was an accomplishment.

Relieving Tensions

Creative fun and breaking the routine is vital for fathers, too, who can get so busy coping that they forget to make time for entertainment.

Usually there was someplace our daughter could go for the weekend, which would leave us alone. So what I would do is go out and get a pizza or crabs or something like that and bring them into the bedroom and we'd watch movies and "eat out" just like you would do if you were on a date. We did the same thing, we just did it at home.

*

Once a week, I'd go to the grocery store and I'd get groceries, but I'd also go to the florist and get some flowers. I thought, She's lying there in bed all the time and she's got to have something new to look at.

*

I would go out on Saturday and come home with a bag of treats, things that she could have—a new novel or a sponge for taking baths. It was just little things that we could share together on Saturday night. Sometimes we would go out on a fantasy date. It was very important to both of us to escape to this fantasy of a place that we liked, where we didn't have bad associations.

*

For our anniversary, my wife surprised me with two tickets to a concert by my favorite singer. She got them by mail and put them in a card. I got a friend to go with me and had a great time. I think it was one of those rare times when I was totally distracted from all the bad things going on. I was sorry she couldn't go with me, but it did the job. I was singing for a week.

*

I'm a jogger. I absolutely insisted upon jogging for one hour every day between my office hours and the time that I went home to make supper for Sonia. I jogged and that helped a lot, relieved a lot of tension.

*

The Lamaze class helped. We were working together on anticipating the birth—it put a positive light on what was otherwise a relatively difficult situation.

When She Is Hospitalized

When his partner is hospitalized, a father may have a strong urge or emotional need to take care of her. Since the medical condition is usually an emergency, high-tech medicine prevails. Dad can see himself as helplessly watching from the periphery. He may not recognize the powerful support that his very presence provides.

Somebody had called me at work and said, "Elizabeth's in labor and delivery." I think for me it's got to be quite different from most fathers who have no previous history of all this kind of stuff. I think most of it was a recognition that at the time it was occurring, the baby was going to die or there would be an extremely small chance of survival. So it wasn't like, "Oh, my God, what's going on? I don't know what's going to happen." I knew that if she delivered when she was in labor and delivery, that was going to be it.

Elizabeth was clearly terrified and we spent I guess a week or so in the hospital. It was never clear that she wasn't going to give birth during the time that we were there because we kept going back and forth to labor and delivery. I think a lot of it was knowing what it is to have an infant who is that premature.

*

It was very anxiety producing. I would be at the hospital as often as I could—teach a class and go back in and see her during the evening. It was a lot of running back and forth and it was very tiring.

*

I was scared when my wife was hospitalized and didn't really understand what was going on. I felt particularly inadequate in understanding the medical and physiological problems. I felt I had very little control over the situation.

*

There was one weekend I think neither of us will ever forget. We had a scare and went to the hospital. Her mother called and the apartment answering service said we were at the hospital. She panicked and flew down from New York City, and showed up at the hospital. A nurse said to me, "There's somebody here to see you." And I thought, "Who in hell could be looking for me?" And it was my mother-in-law. When the doctor was convinced that this was nothing serious, we all went home. Then that evening, my mother-in-law and I had a big Chinese meal and watched television. We stayed up very, very late because it was just sort of an emotional reaction to the high emotional pitch during the day. I remember us laughing ridiculously at "Saturday Night Live."

Emotions

Fathers are stuck in an awkward position during bedrest. They need to become the primary support and protector for their mates at a time when they, too, are in a crisis. Fathers experience the loss of their partners' ability to nurture and support them in many of the usual ways.

We used to have an expression, "Don't dwell." Whenever one of us would do that, the other one would say at some point, "No dwelling." It meant no dwelling on the possibility of a child—no thinking about names, no thinking about how we were going to fix up the nursery, what kind of carriage we were going to buy. We had done it [dwelled] with the first pregnancy and it made it all the more extraordinarily painful when the baby didn't make it. It's hard not to dwell, because you're so involved with it; it's consuming every bit of your energy, and yet you're not allowed to think about the end result. But you think about it every single second. When our doctor said, "The baby is viable, now we're going for quality . . . ," then we began to think a bit differently and I allowed myself the luxury of going out and buying books about babies. I began to visit stores and price things, and that was very nice.

*

I was guarded with feelings about the baby. I was instinctively trying not to care too much, then I would catch myself and feel bad. I had to work hard to overcome this.

*

The difficulty, I think, in a lot of this is if you have a sense that the sacrifice is going to produce something, then you have some relative degree of confidence in it. And because there are no guarantees in life, you can't say, "Oh, I can go through this next four months of really horrible things because I know I'm going to have a beautiful baby." You don't sign a contract and nobody's going to promise you anything. You just do the best you can, and if it works out then all this seems to fade pretty quickly.

*

I got into the position of playing a particular role, of a person who was going to be calm and who was going to say everything was going to be okay. . . . That was very difficult, because I had promised Elizabeth all along that with re-spect to Evan everything was going to be okay and it wasn't [first baby Evan died]. So . . . I wouldn't say, "Everything's going to be okay." I would say, "I hope everything's going to be okay." I would try to look at the bright side: "Well, look, it's so many weeks," or, "You went to the doctor and every-thing was okay"—try to shed some positive light on it in that way, but I wasn't so reassuring except in a kind of Pollyanna way.

I think both us were terrified—even after we got past the thirty-two weeks, when we took a view medically that the chances of survival were really very elevated. We kept think-ing, well, the drug is going to produce some side effect—the kid's going to be turned around or something, and when Genna came out, she came out like a normal baby! And we still didn't know until they said, "She's okay." Even the first week after she was born, she had a really minor problem with an elevated bilirubin count [jaundice]. Elizabeth was con-vinced that it was some fatal disease. It took some time to develop a sense that this is a healthy baby and things were going to be okay. I would get up in the middle of the night and poke her to see if she was still breathing.

*

It helped me to think of the future. Even though it sounds corny to say it, I knew, one way or another, love would carry us through.

Role Changes

Dramatic role changes are temporarily necessary in high-risk preg-nancy. Couples are forced to do new things in their relationship and go without old comforts—all at a time when stress is high.

It didn't hurt our marriage at all.

*

I get very irritated when I hear people say, "Oh, I'm sure this must have made you, made your relationship stronger."

No, it didn't make it stronger. Who knows how the relationship would have evolved over all those years if it hadn't been for this—maybe better, maybe worse. There were good things and problems before and good things and problems afterward. I don't think this made our relationship, nor did it necessarily take away from our relationship. I think it added a tension to the relationship that probably any relationship could do without.

*

I wanted some sense of credit—that I was doing things that were appropriate for her and trying to entertain and cook and clean and soothe and all those kinds of things and that there would be other fathers or husbands who wouldn't do that. It was difficult for Elizabeth to switch the focus from herself because, obviously, if you spend twenty-four hours a day having contractions, you're thinking about yourself a lot and what could happen to you and what could happen to the baby. And I think it was difficult for her to get beyond that and to say, "Oh, that's really nice. I'm glad you did that." The kind of positive feedback that you'd get in a more typical relationship became more difficult during this period of confinement.

I think in a nonconfinement situation we really work fairly hard at trying to resolve things at the time they come up. There were some times [during bedrest] when Elizabeth would say things that didn't make any sense. It was kind of an emotional response on her part that she was afraid or she was worried. Instead of trying to force a resolution of some issues I just said, "Okay, you're right," because there were times when she was just not a hundred percent. Then, usually later that evening or the next day, she would say, "Did I really say that?"

The experience was so terrifying for Elizabeth that even though I had feelings and they were quite legitimate, I could only deal with them at certain times, when I could see that Elizabeth was strong enough to deal with them, which wasn't all the time. There were times when I was strong and times when she was strong. Even if I had to be the more nurturing one for a period of however long it was, that was okay, because I was going to get my turn later.

When I needed to talk to somebody about what was going on, I really had to talk to Elizabeth, because she was the only one who was in touch with what was going on. That didn't work all the time.

*

There were arguments and shouts and loud words and so on. There were times when we were pissed off at each other and we yelled and we shouted and did all the things that we would normally do.

*

The hardest thing was being deprived of Sonia for a year— whenever there was a reception or something, I would be there and I would always be there alone and people would ask about it and it seemed as if there was nothing else to talk about. That was very, very difficult—in that sense, it was a very lonely year.

Sex Life

Since certain sexual activities may pose a risk for the pregnancy, couples must often cope with a loss of familiar ways to be close.

You can't exactly have a flaming sex life when one party is in this situation. It didn't make sense, because you were afraid any which way you turned you might damage something.

*

The doctor didn't think it was a good idea to have orgasms after twenty weeks. Then you sort of added this other element, that Elizabeth shouldn't get excited by doing anything that would get me aroused, so it was celibacy. His fear was that orgasm was associated with causing contractions. That was not good. That's a very important part of my relationship with Elizabeth and hers with me. We had a really good sex life while she was pregnant before.

*

We have a whole new sex life after all this. It's better than it was before. We weren't supposed to do anything while she was pregnant, because of the contractions. We sort of got into a routine of giving each other back rubs and even foot massages. Now we still do those things because they're great. Of course, it's also great to get back to sex.

Fathers and Children

Fathers take on a primary role with children, which involves learning some new routines and techniques. This is hard enough under ordinary circumstances, but even more of a challenge with children who are struggling to cope with so much change.

I can understand my wife's being in bed, but what are we going to do about this three-year-old now? My wife obviously can't take care of her. First thing I was concerned with was getting the help we needed. That turned out to be a bit of a process: first thing you do is start looking in the phone book and asking all your friends. Hiring a baby-sitter was a lot of money—more than I could really afford to pay.

*

I knew I was going to be more important as a parent than ever before. This had both positive and negative feelings. The negative was a sense of further burdens and responsibilities at a time when I was trying to cope with our anxieties. The positive was that it allowed me to break some molds I had created for myself as a father. I was more attentive—more sensitive to our daughter's needs.

*

Giving that three-year-old a bath—talk about a trip! That was definitely not my cup of tea, that and entertaining a three-year-old after work hours.

*

Probably three out of five nights a week, I called up my friend who had kids and we'd go see them and that took care of a lot of it and helped me a lot. I went to my parents' house a few times, too—anything to help on the entertainment part. Both my parents and her parents are in the neighborhood. Jan's sisters were in the neighborhood, so Julie would go visit them on the weekends, which would give me a break.

Family and Friends

Dads help to protect moms from unwanted visitors and stressful contacts while encouraging positive connections with the outside world. A father's family and friends need to give him more support than before, even if he has trouble asking for help.

I have a very close friend and we would speak every couple of weeks by telephone. I also have a very dear and close friend at work. He and I would be on the phone every night practically, and those were the two guys who kind of got me through it, and one or two others who would come over and visit and so on. That meant a lot to me. There were times when I was very happy not to see people because I really was tired of answering questions and reexplaining the whole goddamn thing. It was just painful and somewhat of a nuisance to tell the story to people who didn't know it, because every time you tell it, in a sense you relive it.

*

My parents called every day. They wanted to be supportive. Parents can be a real drag if they say the wrong thing at the wrong time, but it's kind of hard to figure out how much to tell them and what to tell them—whether they're going to be worried. But for so many people, parents may be closer than any of your friends in terms of frequency of contact, and they do have a role in this whole network.

*

I didn't feel I could leave Elizabeth, and although people would come over, I tended not to use that as an opportunity to get out of the house. If we had it to do over again I would do that—encourage people to come over so I could leave.

*

Friends would come over on Friday or Saturday night and they would bring prepared meals. . . . It was very thoughtful of them. That really broke up the loneliness. We used to look forward incredibly to those evenings.

Life After Bedrest

The adjustment following bedrest may come as a surprise to fathers, too. Even in the best of situations, there is little break between high-risk pregnancy and the chaos of new parenthood.

I was all ready to take her out right after the baby was born. "Let's go do things!" I said. Jan didn't have a lot of strength, because she hadn't done anything for so long, so she really couldn't do much.

*

The first weeks there was some concern, some anxiety about the fact that Michelle was in the intensive care nursery. But basically we were told that she was healthy and we were very pleased. That was a very good time for us. I remember enjoying those weeks enormously—sort of the payoff for all we had gone through. Even what's supposed to be the terrible time of the feedings and the late nights—it was fine.

We sometimes have to be aware not to treat her too gently—not to avoid discipline because we know how much we wanted her and how much she means to us. We try to give her all the love and attention she needs, and yet we realize that you can't buy a child all the things on the shelf because you're so happy to have her.

I suppose if we did it again, this time it would be even more complicated because of Michelle. On the other hand, she would be such an enormous comfort. No matter what happened with the second child, there's a certain pressure that's relieved. When we went into the pregnancy for Michelle, we felt, "This is it. It's this or maybe nothing."

*

In retrospect, it makes it clear how much we want to have a child. How much, I guess, we are willing to sacrifice or pain we are willing to experience in order to have a child.

23

*

Bedrest and
the Couple

Relationship on a Roller Coaster

If you think of pregnancy as a journey by train, you can see that the track is long but fairly smooth. You can predict the stops along the way and you know where and when you will get off. High-risk pregnancy is a roller coaster. Just when the ride is level and you begin to relax, the car takes a death-defying plunge that leaves you breathless. You are suspended in mid-fall, not knowing when the bottom will come. At the end of the drop, you take a gasp of air, spin two loops upside down, and jerk to a slow, noisy climb back to the top. It all went so fast that you're not sure where you've been, and the finish is entirely unpredictable.

Your relationship with the baby's father is on that roller coaster, too. It would be nice to take the scenic route in a cushioned, luxury train, but you didn't get tickets for that ride. The two of you can hold hands, scream together on the way down, smile in anticipation of the good parts, and feel the relief when it's over. When you're most scared, you can grab each other and make faces. You won't

171

know ahead of time where the track is smooth and where it turns, but at least you aren't alone on the ride.

Getting the News

The news that their baby is at risk hits a couple like a bolt of lightning. Even those who expected some trouble say that there was a period of shock at first. Each parent goes through somewhat predictable phases while absorbing the bad news and learning to cope. If fathers and mothers could move through the stages of coping in tandem, this chapter might not be necessary. Unfortunately, real life is much more complicated! Dad may be terribly concerned about getting all of the medical details and treatment options just when Mom is numb, unable to believe that there is real trouble. Or she may take to her bed on doctor's advice only to have her spouse wonder if she is overreacting in order to avoid housework. In these circumstances, it is up to the spouse who recognizes the medical problem to gently help the other partner recognize the seriousness of the situation.

There will be times when your moods and needs match and times when you are in really different places. One parent clings to hope in an effort to will the baby to survive; the other parent is afraid to hope because hope could lead to disappointment. Maybe you've experienced this already. You wish to be reassured with hopeful words or wish your partner would stop being so damned optimistic. It helps to recognize that everything is topsy-turvy now. Your roles are different, your moods are different, and you experience change from moment to moment. The two of you may part in the morning as a well-matched pair and find by evening that you can't say a thing to each other that is right.

Don't despair! This upheaval is normal, given your situation. A new balance will be achieved once you learn how you each react in a crisis. You will come to appreciate individual strengths and to anticipate weaknesses requiring extra support.

Immediate Arrangements

Couples need to make rapid plans in the first moments and days after hearing the bedrest prescription. This is a time to work together to understand the medical problem, list what needs to be done, and decide who will do what in the days to come. We highly recommend that fathers see the obstetrician with mothers at least once so that they can hear firsthand about the medical complication and treatment possibilities. As a couple, this can be a time of chaos. You are busy making decisions and may well feel a little numb.

Once the immediate plans are in place, reality begins to set in. One partner may express a lot of sadness or anger or look for someone to blame for the problem. Be aware that this is a part of the process of coping with disappointment and loss. Try to listen tolerantly to each other. Attempts to talk anyone out of his or her feelings only lead to frustration and feeling misunderstood.

Over the Long Haul

As you begin to adapt to your new roles, you will find that there is less confusion. Your routines as a couple become fairly clear. It is tempting to expect smooth sailing from here on and to conclude that something is wrong if you keep having trouble.

You probably don't realize how much turbulence there is in routine pregnancy. Dads begin to think about earning potential, life insurance, colleges, being trapped in their jobs, responsibility, lost youth. Moms mourn for their figures, wonder about their sexuality, get confused about work versus home decisions, think pregnancy was a big mistake. Ambivalence and anxiety are normal for this phase of life. It is too easy to assume that all the couples with "normal" pregnancies are just fine. Or to decide that the other bedrest parents do it much better than the two of you. These are faulty assumptions.

You *do* differ from couples in routine pregnancy in the ways that you mark the passage of time. Ordinarily, a pregnancy has a predictable set of developmental milestones and can be counted upon to progress in an orderly way. Couples in high-risk pregnancy

describe themselves as lurching from incident to incident, counting time in days or weeks instead of months. They have less a sense
of accomplishment than a sense of survival.

Mothers and Fathers

Differences in Experience

As your baby develops, you will start to be more hopeful and begin
to anticipate holding your child. You will become preoccupied with
the baby's kicks, hiccups, rolls, acrobatics. How many times have
you seen a pregnant woman sitting in a crowd with her hands on
her swollen belly, her face dreamy, totally distracted by the activity
inside her body? This peaceful scene seems remote from the realities of high-risk pregnancy, but nearing your due date makes it a
possibility for you. Nature has a way of bringing about this internal
focus for pregnant mothers.

Dad, on the other hand, has been working double shifts for too
long. He senses your preoccupation and realizes that you are less
available to pay attention to him. Even though he knows it makes
no sense, he may resent the time you have to lie in bed and think of
yourself.

Like most fathers, he will probably do the majority of his
bonding when the baby arrives. Labor, delivery, and holding the
baby will bring about his attachment. The baby is such a real child
to you, moving about inside you, and more of a potential child to
him. Although this isn't the way that all expectant parents feel, the
pattern is so common that it is considered normal. You can avoid
being overly critical of each other if you accept this difference.

Another difference between you is in the nature of your roles in
this high-risk drama. The mother's body is the focus of intense
emotional energy and professional attention. You are touched by
many people, weighed, measured, probed, questioned. Usually, a
network of concerned people forms around you. You have responsibility for the baby that no one else can duplicate. Whether you
want the job or not, you have landed the starring role in this drama.

Father takes a giant step outward, into the periphery of the play. He builds the scenery, stocks the refreshment stand, straightens up the theater, scrubs the rest rooms, drives the actors to and from rehearsals, watches the director (who clearly knows more than he does), coaches the star, sees the show from behind the curtain, and delivers the bouquet to the triumphant star—all of this without ever taking a bow! Is it any wonder that the man behind the scenes sometimes feels like running away from it all?

Differences in Style

Just as your experiences in this pregnancy are different, your individual styles of coping with stress are likely to be different as well. Since this is a crisis time, the things that you liked and didn't like about each other before are apt to be exaggerated. Differences in style can wreak havoc with your ability to communicate under pressure, but they can also be a blessing, when one person can help the other because the helper has special skills.

Perhaps you are a verbal problem-solver who values talking as a way to handle hard times. Maybe you express your feelings in words, tears, laughs, and shouts. Since you believe that talking and listening make a big difference in your ability to cope, you talk a lot when times are hard and feel helped when someone listens.

This behavior can be very confusing to a man who feels that he is doing nothing to solve the problem if he merely listens to your distress. He would be hard-pressed to understand that his attentive listening and your emotional talking could be all that you need at the moment. If your partner's primary focus is on *doing* things, he is likely to feel that he is not making a contribution unless he is doing something concrete. Rather than listen to your worries, he will try to fix things by suggesting solutions.

Many men cope with their own upset feelings at this time by plunging into a frenzy of activity. In addition to their jobs and the added household responsibilities, they may suddenly decide to build an addition to the house or launch a new project at work. Expectant fathers in general often baffle their spouses by abruptly going into episodes of major "doing."

This is where couples can get into trouble without understanding that each person is making an innocent mistake. She can conclude that he doesn't understand or accept her feelings when he is really trying to help. She can misinterpret his spurt of activity as abandonment when he sees himself as producing more, out of love for his family. He can decide that she only wants to wallow in self-pity when she is actually working on feeling better in her own way. If you notice these patterns in your relationship, take a moment to see if there is a more positive way to interpret your partner's behavior.

So What Can You Anticipate?

There are many ways in which bedrest can change life for you as a couple. The most obvious changes are in the details of everyday life. The division of household tasks has to be revised in a way that generally results in increasing your partner's workload enormously. Often, this is a time of financial hardship. The budget will be stretched by heavy medical bills and wages for house cleaners and baby-sitters. Your social life, leisure activities, and hobbies will be adjusted to accommodate the limitations of bedrest. Just when you might be feeling a strong need for physical closeness, your doctor may recommend that you limit sexual activity. All of this adds up to a level of chronic stress that becomes a familiar but unwelcome houseguest.

Less obvious is the unspoken anxiety—the worry about your baby's survival. You may find yourselves remembering the loss of another baby or having feelings of grief in advance about the possible loss of this child. It is hard to talk about this subject. You can even feel superstitious, thinking that saying the words will make bad things more likely to happen.

What Can You Do?

Think about what you usually enjoy doing. If these things are still possible while you are in bed, by all means do them. Those favorite activities that don't mesh with bedrest can often be adapted to the new situation. Perhaps you both enjoyed yard work. Although you can't tend your garden now, together you can plan a future garden, write for seed catalogues, and care for a few special houseplants at your bedside.

All that is special and unique about your relationship can be a great support as you accomplish the task of protecting your pregnancy. Be very attentive to what is valuable to you about each other and this relationship. This is fuel to get you through the days ahead. Learn what you can about the feelings and needs of your partner; also be as expressive as you can be about yourself. Sometimes people are afraid that telling their feelings will cause pain when, in reality, not knowing what a partner feels or wants can be even more painful. Listen with care, but remember not to take all things said in a moment of anxiety to heart.

Have some fun. Life can get awfully serious right now. Is this how things always are for you? Play a practical joke or two on each other. Play the games that you like, or learn some new ones together.

Don't be afraid to touch each other. This is a time when physical contact is especially important, even if sex isn't a good idea.

What About Sex?

When a doctor advises "no sex," have him or her spell out which sexual activities are risky and which are likely to be okay. You will need a clear opinion regarding what you and your partner can do without aggravating your medical complication. Sometimes when the recommendation is no sex, your doctor means no sexual intercourse; sometimes your doctor is advising you to avoid intercourse and *all* sexual activities that might lead to a woman's orgasm (an orgasm causes the uterus to contract and can raise a woman's blood pressure).

Once you and your partner clearly understand your doctor's advice, do your best to talk openly about your sexual relationship. Giving up intercourse and orgasm does not mean you must give up sexuality. The man's orgasm is not a risk to the pregnancy unless it involves the woman becoming so aroused that she might experience orgasm. You can explore other alternatives for physical close-ness, such as cuddling and massage.

Do allow yourselves to be sexual in ways that you and your doctor consider safe. Many couples get frightened when cautioned against some sexual activities and leap to the conclusion that *all* sexuality is dangerous for the baby. Don't do this to yourselves. Try some of the activities that aren't on your hazardous list, but pay attention to the way your body responds. Talk to your doctor if you have any worries.

During pregnancy, many women and men experience changes in sexual desire. Some individuals are more interested in sex, some less so. Some men feel less desire when looking at their partner's enlarged belly; some find this change attractive. Some women feel more beautiful as they change physically; some feel less alluring as their pregnancy progresses. All of these reactions are normal.

What About Conflict?

Maybe your style is loud and dramatic with door slamming and dish breaking. Or maybe you are quiet and thoughtful, carefully nego-tiating disagreements. These styles can be retained while you are in bed. Perhaps you can't slam doors, but a few strategically placed old dishes next to your bed can certainly be shattered (as long as somebody agrees to clean up after you! Otherwise, use Nerf balls).

Anger is an inevitable, healthy part of every relationship and its expression is a valuable way to relieve stress. Prior to this preg-nancy, you argued with each other. Nothing has changed. High-risk pregnancy does not confer sainthood on either parent. Moreover, it makes sense to feel some anger at the pregnancy and about the enormous difficulty of bedrest. Sometimes each of you might think, Why me? A father may ask himself, "Why doesn't her body work better? . . . Why must she make so many demands all the time?" A mother could say to herself, "He gets to go out every day and I'm stuck here! . . . He's not doing enough to keep things going around the house!" These reactions are normal. Anger and con-structive arguments give you a valuable opportunity to talk about how the two of you are handling day-to-day life during bedrest.

For a few mothers on bedrest, expressing anger in the normal fashion may cause increased contractions or raise their blood pressure. In these situations, it is best to find another way to deal with anger. Some couples write notes to each other about areas of disagreement; some find distracting activities to take their minds off anger. A father might take up a vigorous exercise program. There are times when it may be best to let conflicts go unresolved; not all problems have to be solved today.

The Father's Feelings

The baby's father has a difficult role, which is made even more difficult by the great increase in his work load. Friends and family may not appreciate the emotional burden he carries. As a bedrest father, he can become overwhelmed trying to do housework and child care in addition to his usual job. He probably feels tired and worried about the baby. He may feel helpless because, in spite of all of his hard work, he can do nothing that will guarantee the healthy birth of his child. Many men are extremely concerned about their partner's health. Some men in this situation become physically ill from stress, lack of sleep, and lack of exercise.

A father is often encouraged to be strong. He is asked by others how his partner is doing rather than how he feels. In fact, he is asked about his own health and feelings so little that he may begin to think that he must keep his needs and frustration to himself. Perhaps he may feel that he is being pressured to be a superman who does everything and leans on no one. He can worry that talking to his partner about his own feelings could be too much of a burden for her. He may feel awkward letting his friends know about his concerns, but only by doing so can he get the support he needs.

Your partner must spend some time taking care of himself so that he will have the emotional and physical energy to do the things he needs to do while you are in bed. He may feel guilty about going to a movie or a gym or just spending an evening with friends while someone else is at home with you. Remind him that he needs this time away; the benefit to both of you will be worth the inconvenience.

The Mother's Feelings

The mother feels the tug of trying to attend to her own needs while worrying about her baby and the needs of her partner. As part of the couple, you may feel less valuable because you now need so much done for you and you are unable to make a number of your usual contributions. You, too, can have your secret feelings. You may feel anger about your dependency, shame about the way your body is functioning, sadness about the strain on your partner, and fear that you are asking for too much. You may resent his relative freedom and fear his rejection. When your sex life is seriously limited and your home life is chronically stressful, you can begin to worry that he will find a more enjoyable woman somewhere else. You may want to be able to listen to your partner but find yourself impatient and unsympathetic when life is not going well for him. If he comes home and complains about the delay in the train, the cold weather, or some aggravation at his job, you may find yourself resenting his ability to go out into the world and experience all of this. Or you may become overly critical of yourself as a spouse, not appreciating that taking care of your baby leaves you with very little emotional reserve.

It can be so hard to give up your usual role that you may be tempted to criticize your partner's efforts to fill your shoes. You'll notice that he buys a different brand of spaghetti, straightens up once a week rather than once a day as you did, feeds the kids on a different schedule. Tread gently here. Some things are important and need to be negotiated; many things are not so important. Some of your criticizing may be a way of letting off steam about not being able to do things yourself. Hooking a rug, throwing a beanbag, talking to a friend, arranging a daily fifteen-minute complaining time—these things can ease the frustration.

In spite of your physical limitations, there are things that you can do to support your relationship. Order your partner's favorite take-out meal, get him a book or gadget from a catalogue, order tickets for a play or concert, plan a date night at home with candles and fancy clothes, rub his back, ask a friend to take him out for an evening, play his favorite music, or send a funny card to his office.

Teamwork

If you can focus your efforts on working as a team during your pregnancy, you will find it easier to get through the obstacles that bedrest presents. Together, you can figure out how you will share tasks and what kind of help you need from others. Teamwork is the feeling that you're in this together and will do what needs to be done. You can take care of meals as a team if you plan menus and make shopping lists, and he goes to the store. You can work together on medical care by going as a couple to some of the appointments and talking about the treatment options. You can compare auto repair prices by phone; your partner can deliver the car. You can sort laundry; he can wash it. You can find a childbirth educator who makes house calls; he can learn to coach childbirth. Just as you can be a team on the tasks, you can team up to plan your entertainment and social life, too.

Take stock of your emotional needs as well as the practical ones when you make your plans. Be sure to seek the support of family and friends. You can help yourselves a great deal if you will be very specific in what you ask people to do for you. They may have no idea when you want a long conversation and when you would prefer a casserole.

And what do you get for all of this effort? You get fathers who know more about household tasks and feel closer to the children. You get men who are better at leaning on friends and at understanding just what their partner usually does at home. You get mothers who can share responsibility for the household and give up trying to be Supermom.

When Teamwork Fails

Since all relationships have their weaknesses, you can predict that these areas will look even worse under the strain of bedrest pregnancy. This is not the time to evaluate the future of your partnership. You may let each other down in small ways or be a major disappointment to each other. Some perfectly loving men and women fall apart in a crisis, but this is not a reason to pack your bags. Give yourselves a chance to be human with human shortcomings.

However, serious conflict can be very frightening when you are confined to bed and so dependent on the assistance of others. Not all pregnant women are involved with supportive men. If your partner refuses to help or acts abusive, be sure to get outside support. Let people know what is happening to you. Don't go without help or protection because you are ashamed to talk about your situation. In some situations, the mother no longer has a relationship with the baby's father. If this is the case for you, you will still need to find people to be on your team, be they family, friends, professionals, or strangers who volunteer to help.

If you and your partner are worried about the way you are coping or feel concerned about the state of your relationship, think about seeking professional help. Ask your doctor, nurse, social worker, or local mental health association for a referral to a licensed mental health professional who is willing to make home visits. Problems needn't be severe to respond to counseling.

Finally

All roller-coaster rides end, no matter how many loops, drops, climbs, or spins there are in the track. There were some points in the trip when you wished you had never bought the ticket. You said, "Why did we think this was a good idea?" Now, at last, with wobbly legs, the two of you stand up and leave by the exit. As you go, you see other eager couples waiting to begin the trip, apprehensive about the adventures ahead. The two of you feel like wise old veterans. Your legs aren't strong, but they kept you in balance during the ride. You leaned on each other to cushion the bumps, and now you lean together so you won't fall down. Maybe you won't take that ride again, but there were some special thrills at the top, you were braver than you expected, and it feels great to be back on solid ground. You made it!

24

*

Mothers' Stories

Many women in bedrest pregnancies feel as if they become a magnet for tales of pregnancy complications. Suddenly, everybody knows a story about someone who was on bedrest. Family, friends, and strangers (including other women in the waiting room of your doctor's office) are eager to swap stories. You may hear "old wives' tales" or a true story that was distorted by the storytellers as it was passed from woman to woman.

By including these real stories of bedrest in the book, we hope to show the variety of personal reactions and coping strategies that mothers adopt. You may find some of these women's stories almost painful to read and at the same time very accurate.

You might read a story and think, "That sounds just like me!" Some other descriptions may be very different from your own situation or feelings. Your family members might also appreciate reading about other bedrest experiences in order to understand more about the impact of this change on you.

In this first story, Diane tells about her introduction to bedrest:

I'll never forget hearing the news that I would need to be on bedrest. Even though I knew that I was at risk for preterm labor, I had never really thought of bedrest. After my doctor stitched my cervix, he said that I had a lot of effacement and that he wanted me to stay in bed for a week. My husband and I scrambled to get help but found no relatives or friends who were able to come assist me with our three-year-old. Just by coincidence, a secretary in my husband's office was unable to type due to a broken finger. She offered to take the job.

It was so anxiety provoking to lie there waiting for the potential contractions that could signal the end of my pregnancy. I found it hard to be in bed in the presence of a woman I had only known from office parties. I really wished that someone else would schedule the days, organize the meals, and give directions to my helper. It felt uncomfortable to have a paid attendant.

As if all of this weren't enough, my husband was scheduled to speak at a conference halfway across the country. I had one huge contraction on the morning of his flight. Neither of us knew what to do. In the end, we decided that he should go to the conference and keep in touch by phone.

I was up in one week feeling terribly proud that I had survived a week in bed. Later I learned that my doctor planned for me to begin bedrest again at twenty-nine weeks as a preventive measure. Looking back on the experience, I came to appreciate that even the news of very brief bedrest can be a shock.

Cheryl describes the events of a six-month bedrest with two small children at home. In spite of the many obstacles, she managed to retain a sense of humor:

Within two months of moving [to a new city], I discovered I was pregnant. Relying upon my past experiences, I quickly located an obstetrician, anticipating a fourth miscarriage. I remember hoping that it would be soon because the longer the pregnancy continued, the more complicated and frightening the miscarriage would become. In addition, I was very concerned about finding temporary care for my two daughters, then ages sixteen months and three years (my husband and I had adopted our daughters from Korea), in case I had to enter the hospital.

When after twelve weeks I did not miscarry, I switched obstetricians to a group with experience in high-risk pregnancies. At my first visit, I filled the doctor in on my long and involved medical history—I'm a DES daughter (congenital uterine and cervical abnormalities); infertility; three miscarriages; three D&Cs; uterine fibroid; over age thirty-five. She recommended a cervical cerclage [strengthening a weak cervix with stitches] in order to prevent another miscarriage.

At the end of my fifteenth week of pregnancy, the cerclage was performed. I had already begun to dilate and my doctor later told me she didn't expect the cerclage to hold. As I awoke from the anesthesia, my doctor informed me that I would have to begin complete bedrest immediately. I agreed, not having the foggiest notion what I was agreeing to. . . . I realized that I was in a new home, in a new place, with two small children, no support system, and my doctor had instructed me to stay in bed except for visits to the bathroom. My mother-in-law agreed to stay while I frantically began the process of hiring a full-time babysitter. I contacted five agencies and called every name they gave me. After what seemed like a hundred calls, we contacted a young woman in Iowa who seemed promising. We had our nanny after four weeks of searching.

For eight weeks I endured bedrest at home. I hated being on the periphery of the activity at home, relying on others for everything, and seeing my children intermittently throughout the day. The house was, to put it mildly, less than organized. My husband was coping with the stress of a new job, additional child care and home responsibility, concern for our unborn child, and an increasingly crazed spouse. I fought a daily battle with myself over the cleanliness (or lack thereof) of my room and bathroom. I am a compulsive type and it took all my resolve to refrain from wiping, mopping, and/or scrubbing. I didn't think things could be any worse—I read three newspapers a day cover to cover, watched every talk show going, and stared at the walls and carpeting of my room vowing I would change them dramatically the minute I was up and about. The high points of this period were the phone calls from my Confinement Line volunteer Liz, my daughter's fourth birthday party (she opened gifts in my room), and the day my mother-in-law set fire to my kitchen (as alarms blared and a fire truck screamed up the street, my daughter repeatedly ran upstairs and down to assure me Grandma had it all under control).

At my scheduled visit during week 24, my doctor determined I was dilating and in danger of having the baby at any moment. She immediately signed me into the hospital. I remember how upset I was to have to go out into the doctor's waiting room to tell my daughters I would unexpectedly not be going back home with them that day.

My forty-nine-day stay at the hospital began the day before New Year's Eve. My New Year's extravaganza included viewing an exciting round of professional wrestling on TV (my roommate was a fan), and a glass of cranberry juice. My husband had an even more exciting time at home wrestling with a broken water main that caused a rather spectacular geyser in the middle of our front yard. In addition, our health insurance company called my husband at 8:00 P.M. New Year's Eve to inform him they would pay for me to stay in the hospital for two days maximum rather than the fifteen weeks recommended by my doctors. This conflict raged on for the first two weeks of my hospital stay. Finally the insurance company agreed to cover the cost of my stay after my doctor quoted costs associated with the birth of a premature infant and my husband's company threatened to switch to another insurance carrier. (Ironically, the insurance company later used a description of my case history to demonstrate cost-efficient case management in their company newsletter).

While in the hospital, my bed was positioned so that my head was lower than my hips to minimize the pressure on my cervix. For forty-nine days I was not allowed out of bed for *any* reason. This was the bottom for me. The nursing staff was great—they took me through the Lamaze techniques and stopped by to chat when I couldn't sleep in the middle of the night—and I had plenty of visitors, but this was the hardest thing I have ever done in my life. If only someone could have assured me that by following all directions a positive result could be guaranteed! Instead, I spent months concentrating like a maniac on every twinge and ache, sure that disaster was just around the bend.

During week 27, I went into labor. My doctors were able to stop it with medication. For these weeks, nurses monitored my pulse and blood pressure and the baby's heart rate every four hours around the clock (not conducive to a good night's sleep). Once a week I was wheeled into Labor and Delivery for a nonstress test.

At week 30 my doctors allowed me to go home, on bedrest, for the rest of my pregnancy. At home I used a home monitor to alert my doctors to any increase in my uterine activity before the situation could reach a crisis point. Twice a day I hooked up the monitor for thirty minutes and then sent the results over the phone line to a nurse at the other end, who would then interpret the reading. On the three occasions when my uterine contractions surpassed the baseline established by my doctors, the nurse, in conjunction with my doctor, increased my medication and continued to monitor my contractions until I was back below the baseline.

In week 34 my cerclage was removed, and naturally nothing happened. During week 36, my doctors were concerned with the results of my nonstress test and decided to induce labor. After twelve hours, it was determined that the

baby was in the breech position and a Cesarean delivery
was required. On April 8, 1988, Victoria Blair was born, a
robust and healthy seven pounds, four ounces.

The following excerpts from Elizabeth's pregnancy journal
show the intensity of a high-risk pregnancy after a loss. Elizabeth
and David's first child died of complications from prematurity. In
this second pregnancy, Elizabeth spent fourteen weeks in bed and
delivered a healthy baby at thirty-six weeks. Her husband, David,
contributed to Chapter 22, "Fathers' Voices":

October 10

I am 22½ weeks pregnant. I'm supposed to meet Martha for
lunch at noon, but decide to go to a close-out sale at 10:00. It is
a madhouse and by 10:45 I am burned out, having purchased
nothing. To kill time, I walk to the National Gallery, intend-
ing to browse there until lunchtime. On the way, I notice
intermittent but regular pressure on my bladder and I think
that something is wrong. I cancel lunch, go home, and lie
down for the rest of the day. The pressure seems to have gone
away. When David gets home from work he chastises me for
not calling the doctor and I promise to do so tomorrow.

October 11

In the late morning I call the doctor's office to report the
events of yesterday. I assure the doctor's assistant that I'm
not currently experiencing problems, but she tells me, after
consulting with the doctor, to come in and be monitored.

I cancel lunch plans and drive to the hospital. Once
there, I am installed in a labor room and hooked up to a
monitor that measures uterine contractions. The nurse asks
if I can feel anything. I can't, but the monitor shows regular
uterine irritability, which, after an hour or so, changes to
regular contractions.

I am admitted to the hospital and beginning to feel panic. The nurse calls David and tells him not to worry. He comes in another hour. David and I are terrified and talk and hold hands till about 11:00 P.M. . . . .

October 12

I stay in the labor room all day, just for monitoring. They stop the magnesium sulfate in the late afternoon and send me to the antepartum unit. We ask for a single room but they have none available, so they give us a double with an empty bed. It's great to be out of the labor room.

October 13

Contractions begin again late in the morning—back to the labor room for a new I.V. (they had just taken the old one out) and a Ritodrine drip. Before they start it, I resist strenuously and have my first real crying episode since coming to the hospital. I just want to go home. I want the nightmare to go away. I don't want to lose another baby, but I've heard so many bad things about Ritodrine's side effects that I'm terrified.

The resident gives me a little dose of reality and tells me I may go into full-scale labor without it. Of course, I relent. David is very supportive and I don't want him out of my sight. The Ritodrine is awful. My heart rate goes up to 106. I feel disoriented and removed and cannot concentrate. David tries reading to me but I have no idea what he's saying. I feel I'll be psychotic if I have to take it for long. However, the contractions stop.

October 14

After a very restless night, they send me back to the floor. We get a roommate. . . . For David and me the lack of privacy is extremely difficult. We are still grieving for Evan [baby who died] but feel constrained with others around. I also think I'm more anxious having someone else there.

Today I used the bedpan all day, which is fine. I'm terrified of getting up and bringing on more contractions.

October 15

The garbage trucks outside awaken us at 5:30. . . . After all the interruptions of the night and little sleep, we are awakened at 6:00 A.M. to get on the scales. Then at 6:30 a medical student comes by. Then at 7:00, the residents. I'm exhausted. I know I'll get more rest at home. My shower today felt wonderful (especially washing my hair), but late in the afternoon my contractions begin again and it's back to the labor room and I get another I.V. (two pokes this time, and I'm becoming less and less brave). . . . After an hour the contractions stop, but David spends the night anyway. I couldn't do this without him. One of Evan's old nurses is my night nurse and I feel really safe with her and David there. Some of the other nurses are so efficient but remote. I need so much support now.

October 17

Another of Evan's nurses comes by at 6:30 A.M. and holds my hand while Donece tries to draw my blood in the dark so as not to wake up David. We laugh hysterically. If only Donece and Kate could take care of me—the impersonality of the hospital experience is the worst part and I really need to feel as though someone cares. My doctor comes in and stands at the foot of the bed against the wall so I have to crane my neck to look at him. He is cold and unsympathetic (he also delivered three babies last night). Later I cry and tell David I'm hurt because the doctor doesn't care about me.

October 18, 19, 20

The contractions are only minor and I don't tell the nurse till after they're over because I'm determined to stay out of the labor room. On Friday night we drink champagne to celebrate making it through the week. I find I'm quite ambivalent about visitors (and the telephone). I love the attention and caring, but I sense that I get more excited and have more contractions.

October 21

I am sprung! David comes to get me around noon and packs all my stuff. I am ecstatic and terrified. Just in the ten days' time since I've been in the hospital, the leaves have turned and are a beautiful assortment of colors. I feel as though I've been in a mini-time warp. I guess it's nothing like the one I will feel when I finally get out of bed and have this baby.

Penny and Hope, my sister and her daughter, arrive by plane in the evening. It's good to see them.

October 22–24

It's wonderful having Penny here, but Hope is a bit trying. She's hit the terrible twos. Penny cooks and cleans and rearranges the kitchen and hangs the pictures in the bedroom. Our new king-size bed arrives and is beautiful. The cable TV people come to install cable in the bedroom. It's so nice to get the room comfortable and pretty. It will be my lair for many weeks to come—hopefully. The bed is like an aircraft carrier and David seems far away, but I need the space to flail about with all my pillows. I seem to need so many.

A friend stops by with her three-year-old. The little ones become rambunctious. I feel as though I want to ask them to leave but feel awkward about it at the same time. In the evening I have lots of contractions and blame it on visitors.

When Penny and Hope leave on Friday I have mixed feelings. I'm so grateful to Pen for all she's done but I relish the quiet.

October 25

I called my doctor to discuss a possible alternative to going in to the doctor's office for a visit. . . . He is adamant about my coming in to the office without giving good reasons for rejecting my alternatives. I continued to argue and tell him I was terrified of getting out of bed since simply taking a shower seems to bring on contractions. He finally tells me I am "high-strung." I scream, "I am not high-strung," and demand an explanation. He talks about my being aggressive, hard-driving, etc. I get myself so worked up in my anger that I have contractions for two days.

October 26–28

David is a whirlwind of activity and I feel I hardly see him at all. He does a million errands (all for me), cleans the house, and strips both bathrooms of wallpaper. I somehow manage to feel neglected. I feel so insecure because of my helplessness and need constant reassurance. . . .

October 30

I feel helpless when the doorbell rings repeatedly and I can't get up to answer it. . . .

Friends bring a wonderful dinner. I am really overwhelmed by the caring and generosity of spirit of the people I know. Everyone is pitching in to help out in some way. It is still hard for me to tell anyone what needs to be done. I seem to leave it up to people to do what they want. Why can't I just say, "Can you bring dinner for Tuesday night?"

November 1

A real blue day. David is short with me in the morning when I ask for rye toast instead of pumpernickel. He hurls the bread across the room toward the wastebasket. I burst into tears. My feelings of dependency and helplessness are so raw. I cringe at being a burden and fear that's what I'm becoming to David. He's been so wonderful, but there's so much pressure on him. Later in the day, I have an attack of missing Evan and sob again. In the evening, the contractions are really strong and I'm terrified. David tries to be sweet but I'm still feeling hurt from this morning. . . .

January 15

Genna is born! Our beautiful Genna. She lets out a little cry and then is taken by the doctor after being suctioned.

After a while they give her to me and she sucks at my breast, but I am in tremendous pain and it is difficult to feel bonded with her. Then David holds her while I get sewn up. . . . I do breathing and relaxation and hold David's hand, but the pain is so sharp it makes me shudder. I am also shivering with cold. Finally, they finish and put us all back in the family room. For the first time, I feel a sense of being a little family with David and our beautiful little girl. Genna is a gorgeous, darling little one and I feel so lucky to have her.

Bedrest memories are not all painful to recount. Judy tells the delightful story of an uninvited visitor:

I'm not normally afraid of mice. Every spring in our house, we get mice. They're always in the basement, though. They never came up on the first floor, except when I was on bedrest. . . .

I'm lying in bed, all alone in my house, and this mouse

appears in our bedroom and starts running laps around my bed. I just couldn't believe it! I'm just frantic. Is it going to climb up the covers on top of me or how can it get to me? It was just driving me nuts! I had a shopping bag of paperbacks that this friend of mine had given me when I was in the hospital. I started flinging these paperbacks at this mouse and it just kept doing laps. It would hide for a while and then come racing out, and I'd fling a paperback. Finally, I got fed up because I was such a nervous wreck. I said, "I'm going to trigger this labor and I'm going to be in worse shape." I called my husband and said, "You've got to come home and do something about this mouse because it's driving me nuts!" So he comes home and the room looks like a war zone. He walks in the door and there are books and papers, anything that was in my reach that I could throw was thrown all over this bedroom and this mouse is still running laps around the bed. My husband chased the mouse for two or three hours. He was running up and down the halls behind this mouse. He'd think he had it trapped and it would go racing into another closet or into another room. Finally he cornered it in the bathroom and killed it. It was all of an inch or two long. It was this tiny little field mouse. While I was sitting there in bed, it looked like it was about four feet long, 350 pounds. . . . It just took on these enormous proportions . . .

My husband had to go back to work and I didn't want to be alone in the house because I was afraid that the mouse's "relatives" were all going to come to terrorize me for having their little mouse killed. A friend of mine came over and stayed with me. Then I was finally okay and figured that I could survive, that no mouse relatives were going to come to wreak their revenge on me!

Children sometimes seem to run around their mother's bed like that mouse, full of mischief and out of reach. Let's hear from Jeanne:

My three-year-old was frustrated about Mommy always staying in bed and came up with many creative attempts to move me. In one of our rare afternoons alone together, she grabbed the forbidden scissors and looked at me with a gleeful look. When I asked her to give me the scissors, she began to walk around my bed just beyond the reach of my arm. What to do? I tried all of my best persuasive techniques. When those failed, I sank to offering various bribes and finally got openly angry. No luck! As I boiled in frustration, worry, and indecision, she put the scissors down and found something else to do.

Another time, when she was clearly needing a way to express her feelings, my daughter got inventive in the bathroom. When our helper was busy with some housework, my daughter covered her own body with Vaseline from head to toe. She was quite a sight as she proudly displayed her artwork! I felt grateful, for once, to be unable to get out of bed to take care of the problem.

Vicki's son was born at thirty weeks. When he was four years old, after two miscarriages, Vicki began the pregnancy described below. She was on bedrest for over twenty-six weeks due to preterm labor. Her healthy daughter left the hospital on the same day that Vicki did.

February 2

Sixteen weeks pregnant, home on complete bedrest. . . . I'll probably be on bedrest until due date—July 10. This is much earlier and harsher than the predicted, "Take it easy from twenty-four weeks on" that I heard at the start of this pregnancy. I've resigned my job and don't know how we can possibly afford to have any kind of help with housework or child care without my income.

February

People have rallied. Its a funny thing—parents of Lucas's classmates, whom I do not know, have offered rides to and from preschool, have brought food, have come to clean; yet others I know better, I don't hear from at all. It's so tough to ask for help. People make blind offers—"call if I can do anything"—I don't know if they are sincere or not. We are also talking about five months of this and I don't want to use up my offers. Many people say they will take Lucas, but he doesn't know them and he's feeling reluctant to be away from me, even to go to familiar places. He's having a hard time leaving for school two mornings a week. The days last forever. . . .

March–April

We've worked out a routine of two hours of "Sesame Street" a day—gives me the chance to read myself. We are having to do lots of crafts! Kirby has set up the living room into our pregnancy-in-bed room. Lucas has his table and chairs and a movable stack of crafts, games, and snacks on wheels. We are doing lots of imaginative play and I keep thinking this is my chance to really spend quality time here. On the other hand, I sometimes feel if I see any more glitter spilled onto the carpet that I can't clean up, I will absolutely scream!

The medication I'm taking makes me really nervous and hyper and I feel so lonely sometimes. Everyone is so busy. People don't take the time just to come hang out. I could sure use some of that.

Kirby is in school, finishing up in May. He is busting his buns. . . . He works until 5:30, runs home, gets supper, runs to school, and gets home at 10:30 twice a week. Then on weekends he disappears for four or five hours of studying. I make lists of what's most important in terms of housework, but it all seems important to me and he's not here to even see the mounds growing and piling up. I feel resentful that he's continuing his schooling this semester. He wants to be done when this baby arrives, but I need him at home now. I can appreciate that he's on a roll. It just doesn't help the house get clean or help me from feeling so lonely.

I made arrangements to have Lucas at a baby-sitter two mornings a week. I'll have to drive him there, but it's only a few blocks away. I took him there and the baby-sitter's nine-year-old was home from school because he was sick! I couldn't believe that knowing my situation, she didn't call to tell me Lucas would be around a sick child! So much for that. I'll just keep him at home.

Weeks 24 to 30 are really tough for me. I'm scared of having a baby now for I know all the many things that can go wrong. It motivates me. I realize if the baby comes early, every week I could have been lying on the couch, I will be sitting in the intensive care nursery with a preemie.

People continually say to me, "I'd trade places with you. I'd love to lie on the couch for a few weeks." These "few weeks" will be twenty-four at the end, if we make it, and there is no guarantee we will. It's like nursing along a serious illness, but you're not sick.

32 weeks:

In my mind we have made it! We will probably get a baby out of this. A sense of relief that I can't describe. Kirby finished school. He's done. He made it! I'm determined to make it and bring this baby home.

35 weeks:

I had two baby showers. I felt like a normal person. It was absolutely wonderful.

37¹/₂ weeks:

I'll have a C-section at 11:00 A.M. I'm nervous about the C-section and can't believe we actually made it to this day. We'll name her Casey Alison. . . . Casey means brave and surely any child willing to try and come through my body into this world is brave. . . . Kirby is beside me and again the wait seems so long. But finally, finally she's here. . . . She's gorgeous! Our nurse explains to the staff how hard we've worked for this one and I would like to see her if possible. They wrap her up and *hand her to me*. I have her and she's healthy and we did it!

Casey came home with us five days later. I broke down in tears when the doctor told me she was released to go home. We dressed her up and her dad, brother, and I took her home. We folded up the egg-crate mattress and slowly got our lives back together. We certainly feel we are fortunate to have a good outcome and now have a beautiful little angel at our house. I look back at bedrest time as one of the challenges of my life. Few challenges have the potential for such a wonderful outcome. You have to remember that every day, sometimes every hour!

Mothers who have extended hospitalizations develop creative ways to adapt to their new environment. Ann, a veteran of fifteen weeks bedrest, including ten weeks hospitalization for placenta previa, wrote this moving account of her pregnancy:

This was to be my fifth pregnancy. I did have a healthy four-year-old daughter but had suffered three miscarriages at approximately twelve to thirteen weeks gestation. I began to wonder what in the world was wrong with my body that would allow it to eject my own babies. I felt that surely my womb must be an inhospitable place. . . .

After weeks of resting at home, I awoke at four o'clock one morning in a pool of blood. My husband and I quickly headed for the hospital, where I was monitored for a day. At this time a partial placenta previa was diagnosed. I was sent home with orders to stay on "strict bedrest," which specified that I could get up to use the bathroom and to take one shower a day. My doctor kindly and gently explained what I could expect and then added, "Now you'll get to lead the life of a queen." Somehow, I felt less than regal.

After five weeks of conscientious and uneventful bedrest at home, I awoke again at four o'clock in the morning in the middle of a bleed. I was twenty-seven weeks pregnant and terrified. I was hospitalized and once again the weeklong vigil of trying to stay on my left side. Initially, I felt relief rather than devastation at the prospect of being hospitalized for the duration of the pregnancy. The hospital seemed the safest environment for assuring the survival of my baby should a massive bleed occur. It was becoming harder to live with the uncertainty of when or to what extent the previa would strike. I felt that I was living with a time bomb inside of me.

I experienced a range of emotions during my ten-week hospitalization. At times I felt appreciative and content; at other times, feelings of impatience, boredom, and great loneliness emerged. At first I was almost overcome by gratitude at having so many of my basic needs anticipated and addressed. It was as if by magic that meals and snacks appeared—I didn't need to utter a request to anyone! After months of being so dependent on those around me, I was relieved to feel less like a "burden."

Hospitalization helped to alleviate the feelings of isolation which accompany confinement. In the antepartum unit I was surrounded by others like myself; in this environment bedrest was the norm! I was granted an instant and extensive support group. As we shared our test results, hair dryers, magazines, socks, setbacks, hopes, and fears, a strong sense of camaraderie developed among us. Sometimes we stayed awake half the night talking. Sometimes we immersed ourselves in knitting and crocheting projects. At other times, we would lie around like beached whales, complaining bitterly of the trials of our situation and of how we couldn't stand the sight of "regular" pregnant women.

The hospital nurses played an important part in easing our anxiety and despair. They were instrumental in acquainting patients with each other for mutual support. Their stories of veteran antepartum patients offered us encouragement. The nurses were often our advocates, providing suggestions for modifying some of the more restrictive hospital policies that made life difficult during our long-term stays. It was from the nurses that I learned of wheelchair privileges, write-in menu requests, and creative therapy. Most meaningful were their many generous personal touches—magazines brought in from their homes, offers to pick up items for us on their way to work, and frequent visits to chat when they could.

The hospital offered an environment in which I could feel "safe" and be among others like myself. However, a peculiar kind of torture accompanied living through ten stressful weeks with no time or place to be alone. Privacy was simply not a feature of the hospital environment. I had no control over many facets of my day; my desire to take a nap could easily be thwarted by a roomful of anybody's visitors. Phone calls, needlework, and sleep were often interrupted by the nurses' rounds. In such a "social" setting, I felt a need to remain cheerful. I reserved tears for my one sanctuary of privacy—a daily shower.

The prolonged separation from my husband and daughter was the most difficult aspect of my hospitalization. I grappled with trying to justify the security of the hospital environment at the expense of our family's connectedness. The hospital was approximately an hour from our home. Although my husband visited daily, it seemed that we were capable of exchanging only pleasantries. I felt guilty that he was being forced to absorb total responsibility for maintaining the house and for our daughter. He felt overwhelmed. There was so much emotion locked inside both of us, but no setting existed to facilitate its expression.

Hospital visits with my four-year-old daughter were inevitably a disaster. She was suffering from our separation and from having each day full of transitions from caretaker to caretaker. Justifiably, she was angry that I had "abandoned" her for hospital life and a new baby. It was impossible for her to appreciate medical explanations for the fact that her world had turned upside down. Promises of Mommy's eventual return were small comfort to the "here-and-now" mind of a four-year-old. She quickly grew weary of the hour-long ride to the hospital. I was so eager to see her and unrealistically tried to cram all that I felt we were missing into our visits.

On May 2, 1985, our daughter Sarah was delivered by a planned Cesarean section at thirty-six weeks gestation. Sarah's orderly and gentle entrance into the world was in sharp contrast to her tumultuous prenatal history. After months of progesterone, ten sonograms, multiple injections of betamethasone, and week after week of bedrest with intermittent bleeds, Sarah arrived, weighing seven pounds, thirteen ounces. The waiting, hoping, and praying were over. We were elated, grateful, and in a state of disbelief.

25

*

Caring for Your Child

If you have one or more children at home, you may be especially concerned about how you can function as a mother when you are stuck in bed. Although the way you care for your child will change, you will be as important as ever as a parent; just as actively involved as you were before bedrest, the only change being in the location and type of activity. Much more energy goes into telephone work, scheduling, and managing volunteer or paid helpers.

Making Decisions

First, you need to decide what assistance will be needed, whether or not to hire help, and how to set up a workable daily schedule for your child. There are as many solutions to these problems as there are families who have to solve them. Some parents get by with little or no help, some rely on day care or school, some hire full-time help, and others send children to live with relatives for a period of time. Schedules vary from the relatively simple to a complex coordination of numerous volunteers and paid caregivers.

We think it works best if children have frequent contact with their mothers (including regular visits to her if she is hospitalized). You and their father will need to evaluate what works best for you. Although most people feel a financial squeeze during pregnancy, it may be necessary to stretch the budget a bit rather than add to the family's stress by trying to get by without badly needed help.

Planning Your Child's Schedule

Organize your child's days, including regular events such as school, day care, special outings with Dad, and activities at home with Mom. It helps both you and your child to arrange for playmates to visit your home with their parents or for friends to take your child out for an afternoon. Encourage older children to participate in setting their own schedules. All ages benefit from the security and predictability of a schedule in such a time of turmoil. Tell each child what the plan is and who can be expected to be responsible for him or her at any given time. It is a good idea to plan ahead for car pools and to find out who can provide occasional transportation.

You need to make plans for emergency child care in case you go to the hospital or to your doctor on short notice. Keep a list of names and phone numbers of people who are available (a long list with plenty of backups). Prepare your child by explaining that you may need to see the doctor very quickly one day. Let your child know who you will be calling for help if that happens.

What Can My Child and I Do Together?

Once practical arrangements are made, the next challenge is that of finding ways to share your child's life while you are in bed. This is not as difficult as it seems. You are unable to participate in former outdoor activities, but you can devise many activities that will be new and entertaining for both of you. Some mothers share meals by having their child eat at a small table placed next to the bed at mattress height. This same table can be used for a variety of activities such as board games, painting, modeling clay, homework, and drawing. There is nothing like sharing a hug in bed or watching a good television show together. This is also a great time to read aloud your child's favorite books or let an older child read to you. You can use your radio or tape player to introduce your child to the variety and joys of music. What about a sing-along?

Helping Your Child When You Are in the Hospital

If you need to be hospitalized, tell your child in simple terms where you will be and why you are going. In an emergency hospitalization, when it is not possible to notify your child in advance, phone home later to explain what is happening. You can keep in touch by telephone, even with a very young child who may not understand where you are. Hearing you sing a song or tell a bedtime story gives reassurance that you are coming back. A young child may also feel comforted if she can take care of something of yours while you are gone. Perhaps she could keep your pillow or nightgown in her bed at night. An older child will enjoy receiving cards or letters as well as phone calls.

Although hospital visits tend to be emotional for both of you, a child is often reassured by the visit. Some mothers give their visiting children small gifts from a goody bag which can be stocked by their father or a friend. If you are able to do so, a snuggle in your hospital bed is good for both of you. To help your child feel at home in your hospital room, let him have space in a drawer where he can store his special things until he visits you again.

Be prepared for some less-than-satisfactory visits during these times. You may want to fill your child with a week's worth of love in a thirty-minute visit. She stands there at the foot of your hospital bed afraid to come closer and begins to whine about going to the gift shop for a treat. This scene is not uncommon, and it is not a sign that your relationship is ruined. Once you return home to your normal routine, lots of individual attention will heal the hurt and put the two of you back in each other's arms.

How Is My Child Dealing with This Stressful Pregnancy?

Many parents ask themselves, "What is this doing to my child?" Children demonstrate in such dramatic ways that all is not well. They cry, suck their thumbs, wet the bed, fight, pout, get anxious about separation from you, break things, yell, wake up with bad dreams. One of us received a call from the preschool teacher when the bedrest baby was one week old. The teacher, who knew all about the pregnancy, felt concerned because the three-year-old seemed to be under stress. Of course she was!

Let's take a look at those troubling behaviors that can make you feel so worried and guilty. First of all, they are normal. All children have their moments when they are overtired, crabby, and naughty. It is easy to assume that every less-than-perfect behavior is a direct result of your bedrest situation. Most pregnant mothers also get tired, feel crabby, and sometimes yell at their children. Don't expect your child or yourself to be a saint.

Young children are likely to show even more of these attention-grabbing behaviors when a new sibling is on the way. Since this is a pregnancy with a lot of stress, your children are going to cope in the best way they can. This usually means acting out their concerns by *showing* their feelings in their behavior. This is their way of adapting to the stress and starting to feel better. It would make more sense to worry about a child who showed no change in behavior under these circumstances.

Will your child be permanently traumatized by the events of this pregnancy? Probably not. As you recover and gradually return to normal life, your child will relax and get on with the adventures of childhood. Children are emotionally resilient; they have the flexibility to recover. They can cope with difficult times if they have love, permission to show their feelings, and time to adjust.

Can I Do Anything to Help My Child?

You may feel sad, irritated, or guilty about changes in your relationship with your child. Fortunately, there are things you can do to help your child cope successfully. Provide structure and stability in areas that you control. Knowing that family ground rules are still the same is reassuring to a child who sees the family changing. You might feel tempted to relax your expectations, since your child is under such stress. Unfortunately, this relaxation of the rules may create more anxiety for your child at a time when consistency could help her feel more secure. Although you are unable to get out of bed to intervene, you can set limits verbally and support your helpers in maintaining them.

You set a tone in your family that greatly influences how your child will make sense of this situation. If you are apologetic and overcome with guilt, your child may decide that he is the helpless victim of something that is your fault. If you are matter-of-fact about the challenge that you all face and you include your child on the family team, he will see himself as a competent survivor rather than a victim. Children of all ages love to be needed and can be given appropriate jobs that contribute to their sibling's healthy arrival.

Helping Your Child Play Out Feelings

A child benefits a great deal from expressing emotions through play and can gain mastery over what is troubling him or her by playing it out. In order to help your child do this, you can borrow some techniques from play therapists. Keep in mind that the most important aspects of therapeutic play are the expression of feelings and ideas by the child in your presence and your acceptance of them without judgment.

Dolls, puppets, clay, and drawing tools are excellent props. You can lie back and watch the action. Show your attention by making occasional comments that describe what is happening. If you avoid criticizing or questioning, you will be surprised to see how soon your child begins to tell you all about his or her feelings through the play. In some cases, there are very few words expressed.

Annie was driving me crazy while I was in bed pregnant. She's like most two-year-olds, full of beans, but she got into some really bad behavior—breaking things and drawing on the walls, to name two. We got some clay one day and Annie must have spent a whole hour punching and squeezing and smashing it next to my bed. She was really good the rest of the day. After that, we played with clay every day.

Children often express relief when they can communicate strong feelings in this protected manner. A four-year-old boy and his mother used family dolls for their play:

(Child puts mother doll in bed and holds child doll.)

CHILD: Get up, Mommy!
MOTHER: The boy doll is saying, "Get up!"
CHILD: The Mommy won't get up!
MOTHER: That Mommy stays in bed.
CHILD: Wah! Wah! Wah!
MOTHER: The boy is crying. The boy is so sad.

When the play is over, you can move from pure observation to more discussion about what took place.

MOTHER: How do you think that boy felt when his mommy couldn't get up?

Move slowly to talking about your own child's feelings and yours.

MOTHER: Maybe sometimes you feel sad, too, because I have to stay in bed.

Remember that a successful play session is often very brief, a matter of a few minutes. It is easy for parents to feel upset about the feelings their child has expressed and to have an urge to try to make it all better. What is harder to appreciate is that the expression of feelings in itself is a release for your child. Don't be concerned if your child is unable or unwilling to talk much about the play. She or he will probably play out feelings over and over during your pregnancy; it is the expression of feelings over a period of time that is beneficial.

Since young children are ambivalent about new siblings and

have trouble telling the difference between fantasy and actual behavior, they can get frightened thinking that their anger is making something bad happen to the baby or to you. They need to be told that their mad feelings can't hurt the baby, that no one's feelings can make bad things happen to the baby or to you.

Your child will benefit greatly from a straightforward explanation of why you are in bed and how you feel about it:

> The doctor says that I have to stay in bed so the baby can grow big enough to be born. It's hard for you and it's hard for me, too. I feel sad when I can't go to the park with you. We can do some fun new things together here in my room. When I get up after the baby is born, you and I will go to the park to play.

Your Older Child

An older child who is able to express his or her feelings and thoughts in words may still have trouble at this time. You might see an increase in hassling with you over clothes, meals, and bedtimes. She or he may stage numerous last-minute crises, such as abruptly announcing that she needs a special kind of shoe for tomorrow's gym class or he has a sudden need for a new record. These "crises" may be events for which you would have dropped everything in the past, but now you are unable to rush out and take care of things. Such demands serve as a test to see if you will stay in bed. They express your child's anxiety and disappointment about your limitations and represent a wish that you would quit lying around if your help was really needed.

Older children may want physical contact with you, but they are less likely to ask for it. You can brush their hair, scratch their backs, invite them to display their collections on your bed. Two of you can share the bed while you discuss the latest trades of baseball cards, cars, or plastic ponies.

Both girls and boys may pick up some odd ideas about childbearing as they observe your pregnancy. This is a natural time to add to their knowledge of sexual development and reproduction.

They need to know that most pregnancies are much less complicated and difficult than yours. Two excellent books written by Lynda Madaras for children approaching puberty are: *The What's Happening to My Body? Book for Girls* and *The What's Happening to My Body? Book for Boys* (Newmarket Press: New York, 1987).

Luckily, older children are more able to sit with you and talk about the worries that underlie their behavior. Many are frightened that their mother may die from medical complications or that their actions and feelings could cause the situation to worsen. There are great fears that openly expressed anger may aggravate the mother's condition. Your child needs to hear—often—that bedrest will not last forever. Your child also needs to know that once the baby is born, the two of you will continue to have a special relationship.

Your Adolescent

Having an adolescent in the house during bedrest can be a mixed blessing. At this age your child can be a wonderful help to you, but beware of putting too much responsibility on a teenager. Adolescents need mothering, too. Your teen may feel guilty about wanting to be with friends, away from all of the tough times at home. He or she could be acting very angry toward you while hiding fears that you will die or be damaged. In the best of times, most adolescents are confused and ambivalent. They have powerful needs for independence from home coupled with the occasional intense desire for your support and attention.

With a tiny developing baby as the focus of your energies, it can be hard to remember that the adult-size teenager needs reassurances, too. Try to find a blend in which the adolescent can provide some necessary help and also have some guilt-free time off. Look for time to chat and for neutral activities such as watching movies and playing games. Take advantage of opportunities to do normal things together like experimenting with new hairstyles or talking about the latest professional ball game. Be sure to keep up with the events in your teenager's outside life. It will help if Dad and your teen can check out of the house each week for some special activity.

The normal questions and curiosity about sexuality that peak at adolescence can't help but be affected by this unusual pregnancy. You can look upon this as another chance to give information, share your values, and calm any fears that pregnancy is always like this.

When Are You Giving This Baby Back to the Hospital?

When a new baby arrives at home—even after the smoothest and most routine pregnancies—other children in the family experience a rocky time adjusting. Although this period may be even worse after a bedrest pregnancy, keep in mind that much of your child's struggle is the normal process all children go through in learning to accept a new sibling. One of the differences that your unusual pregnancy brings about is the degree of disappointment that your child may feel. She has been waiting so long for you to be back on your feet, functioning like good old Mom again. It can come as a shock to discover that you still need a lot of rest and that a new baby is receiving so much of your attention. Your child may not understand that you will get stronger and the baby care will get easier.

As long as there are love and patience, most of the adjustment will be accomplished with the passage of time. You can help your child by spending some time with him alone as often as possible. This lets him know that he still has a special place in your heart.

Some children appear to be deeply disturbed by the effects of a bedrest pregnancy, while others seem to take it in stride. Regardless of the kind of reactions they display, most children manage to cope when they need to and recover well from the stress of a high-risk pregnancy. Many families report positive changes in their family life as a result of their efforts to adapt to this unusual situation. Children and their fathers may form a stronger bond that lasts beyond the pregnancy. Some children feel a sense of pride in themselves for helping out when things were tough. Almost all children learn that there are many people other than Mom who can love and take care of them. This can lead to positive feelings of independence and security.

Although having a mother on bedrest is difficult, your child can develop new self-esteem derived from coping successfully with a major challenge.

26

※

Your Friends

For most women, pregnancy is a change that alters their interests and the way they think about work, family, and friends. When you became pregnant, some things became very important to you and other things became less important. The changes in yourself affected your friendships with the people around you, too.

When your doctor informed you that your pregnancy would require medical management and extended periods of lying down, you underwent even more changes. During the first few days, the immediate stabilization of your medical condition became your most important goal, while all the other things you were doing or had planned to do were pushed out of your mind. Gradually, as you begin to manage your bedrest time, you will notice that you are drawing closer to your doctor, nurse, and other medical staff. You may seek out other high-risk pregnant women and retreat from contact with women who are having routine pregnancies.

How Your Friends View You

Your friends have already been adjusting to your pregnancy. Now, when your friends visit you, they see you lying in bed on a special mattress overlay, propped up by pillows and foam bolsters. You may remind one of a relative who was seriously ill. Another may be planning a pregnancy and feel alarmed.

Be understanding of your friends. Some will be more supportive than others during your pregnancy bedrest. You may be pleasantly surprised at the reactions of some of the people you know; other friends may behave in ways that disappoint you. The key point is that this is not the time to test your friendships. A friend who is unable to be involved with you now may be dealing with personal issues that are intensified when she sees your high-risk pregnancy.

You can help your friends help you by suggesting specific tasks. Let them do the footwork for you—the trips to the hardware store, supermarket, and library. If you are used to trading favors with friends, you may feel guilty that your activities are so limited right now. Some women find new ways to help others, such as phone calling, mending, or taping special television shows. This is terrific if you feel up to it, but coping with your own life may be all that you can do at this time. Remember how wonderful it feels to do a good deed? That special feeling is what you can give to your friends as they give their energy to you.

I was talking to my sister, Pam, one day about how hard it was to keep asking for help, knowing that I could do nothing for those who helped me. I had begun to make an imaginary list in my head of how much I "owed" each person and I thought I would be "in debt" for years to come! Pam responded that she wondered why it was so hard to accept help as a gift. She told me of a time when she had had similar feelings. Early in her marriage, she had a small child and no car available during the day. A faithful friend kept giving her rides and other kinds of assistance. Pam remembered telling her friend, "I'll never be able to return all your favors!" Her generous friend had replied, "No, you might not be able to do these things for me, but someday you'll help somebody else." My sister had reassured me that *my* friends weren't keeping score either. I knew someday that I would be in a position to give to others.

When Friends Visit

As soon as you tell your friends and family that you are on pregnancy bedrest, many of them will want to come visit. Here's a composite of all the nightmare visits pregnancy bedresters have actually experienced:

> She said she would drop by at 3:00 P.M., and was ringing my doorbell an hour earlier. I was still napping, in preparation for her visit, and walked to the door in my nightgown. She handed me her coat, which felt like a ton of bricks, and I walked to the closet to hang it up. Then we walked back into the bedroom and I lay down. As soon as I was settled, she asked if she could have some coffee. I told her where the coffee was and she disappeared for twenty minutes and returned with her own mug. She stared at me and then said I looked better. I asked her if there was any hot water left (hoping for a cup of tea) and she replied, "Now, you know you shouldn't be getting up just to make tea!" Then she made herself comfortable on the bed and began to gossip about our friends at work. She handed me an envelope from my supervisor, which clearly had been opened. Fortunately, about five minutes later, my nurse called. She remained on my bed, listening! My nurse wanted me to perform a home monitoring test, which seemed very exciting for my visitor: she asked if she could watch. I told her it would be best if I could be alone, and asked her if she could see herself out as I needed to settle down before strapping on the equipment. She gave me a look that indicated I clearly had no manners, gathered herself up, left the coffee mug, paused at the door, and said cheerily, "Well, at least you'll be well rested when your baby is born."

When people learn that you must remain in bed, they feel an obligation to express their sympathy and try to cheer you up. In other words, they want to make a sick call. Such sick calls are unpredictable. The person sounds upbeat during the telephone call, arrives with smiles and flowers, and after a few minutes begins to ask you questions about how your medical complication began or tells pregnancy stories of situations worse than yours.

She told me not to worry—my situation was not as bad as one poor woman who had the worst story she had ever heard. Then she began to tell me about that other poor woman. In about a minute, I realized that this worst story was *my story.* She was telling me about all my other pregnancy losses, with a few extras she was making up or someone else had exaggerated. Now, it seems funny. Then, I was speechless with horror and rage.

How do you prevent sick calls? The trick is to plan ahead for your time with visitors. First, discourage surprise visits. When someone offers to drop by next week, explain that you have limited visiting hours, and set a specific date and time that is best *for you.* If you answer the doorbell and find a surprise visitor at the door, thank that person for thinking of you, express regret that you can't have visitors today, and promise to telephone later in the week. Be sure to make that follow-up call, so that this visitor learns that while the good intentions are appreciated, your visiting time has to be planned ahead.

During visits, do something together. Your visitor can help select a pregnancy dress from a catalogue or measure a hem. A friend who does a craft can teach you how to start a project or help you with the finishing touches.

End your visit while you and your friend are both feeling positive. When you've finished watching a movie, or eaten a snack and completed a list of catalogue numbers, it's the right time to thank her for the visit and explain that you need to rest. A trick to moving your friend to the door is to ask her to help you out of bed and walk you to the bathroom. Point your visitor in the direction of the front door and look longingly at the bathroom. In our experience, even the most reluctant to leave got the hint at the bathroom door.

Your Child's Friends and Their Parents

Your child has a circle of friends from play group, school, basketball league, or religious class. You have met these children, and they know you from time they have spent in your home and your car, and seeing you volunteer at school functions. Now your situation has changed and become a bit scary. Your daughter's friend Kathy thinks you are very sick; your son's friend Tom thinks you are now disabled because you can't get out of bed.

Kathy's and Tom's parents may be a bit uneasy with your bedrest situation, too. They may have personal feelings that are intensified when hearing about your bedrest pregnancy. They may be uneasy about their children seeing another parent in her nightgown, or they may confuse your being in bed with being sick and infectious. They may have trouble explaining to their children why you are on bedrest.

You can help your child by defusing the fears of parents. Put yourself in their place and figure out what words would reassure you. It's not necessary to explain the specifics of your medical condition; more important to parents are the limits on your ability to get around the home.

It's understandable that other parents will suggest that your child play in their home. Their offers can be made with the best intentions—to spare you noise and disruption. But you don't want your child to think that your bedrest is the reason your home is off-limits. Suggest that parents stop in for a minute to chat with you when returning your child home. The parent will see you, another parent, wearing pants and a pregnancy top, settled in an orderly room, in a neat home. You will talk about the latest school project or volunteer work. Meanwhile, after a quick peek at you, your child's friend is reassured and probably runs to your child's room.

A note of caution here: if you are preparing for an "I'm-just-lying-down, I'm-not-contagious" visit with a child's parent, don't get out of bed and spend the day cleaning your home. The night before, insist that your child straighten his or her room and the family straighten up the living room. All you should be doing is what you normally would do on bedrest—changing into a day outfit and busying yourself with a craft or a book.

If you have a very young child, you may be part of a play group. It's wise not to host a group of toddlers in your home. Your side table and medical equipment are within reach of small children. Even if you are allowed enough sitting time, the noise, the numbers of parents and children will exhaust you. You might arrange to hire a sitter to take your child to a play group. You can visit briefly with one playmate's mother while both toddlers remain in a playpen.

Sometimes a mother will offer to play with your child and her child at your home. Use visitor-privileges time for this play visit. Even if you remain in your room, you will be participating by answering questions, responding to your child's shouts, and directing the other parent where to find toys, wipes, and snacks. In fact, during a play visit your child may be especially demanding in an effort to demonstrate that her mother is playing, too.

Older children are involved in outside activities and you will need to make an arrangement with other parents for transportation. You could become the dispatcher for a car pool, thus carrying your share of tasks. Or you could simply adjust temporarily to being dependent upon these parents for help. Later in the year, when you are back on your feet, you can offer sleep-overs for your children's friends to give their parents some evenings off from child care.

Your constant presence at home can be beneficial to your teenager. On a weekend night, your teenage daughter can invite a few friends to watch their favorite horror movie. Just being in the home, awake and in earshot (use the walkie-talkies), will discourage any inappropriate behavior. Don't be surprised by respectful and considerate behavior displayed by your teenager's friends. One bedrester claimed that several of her son's friends showed up in her doorway one evening and offered to make her a snack.

When Your Friend Is a Child

You may have a special friendship with a niece or nephew. Or you may be an "aunt" to a friend's child. These children have the same feelings of anxiety about your high-risk pregnancy and bedrest. Telephone calls can be reassuring and you may want to send some homemade postcards. But your young friend may really need to see you to calm his fears. Arrange for a brief visit to do a small activity he likes or share with him a craft or a song you have practiced.

One woman's four-year-old daughter insisted that she and her mother visit me. Her mother was a bit hesitant, but her daughter would not be put off. When my young friend entered my room, she plopped herself on my bed and pulled a small toy out of her pocket. "Here. You need a toy to play with in bed," she declared, and proceeded to teach me how to play. It was the kindest, most heartfelt offer of help I had ever received.

BACK ON YOUR
FEET AGAIN

27

*

Finishing Your
Bedrest

There comes a time in your bedrest pregnancy when your doctor or
nurse begins to talk about childbirth. During an office visit, you are
asked if you are starting to make plans for your baby.

Why Make Plans?

It may seem like an odd luxury in the midst of a high-risk pregnancy to think about making plans to be a mother. Even in a routine
pregnancy, mothers are often so preoccupied thinking about labor
and delivery that they have little imagination left to picture life
with a newborn. "I'll worry about that later!" is a common approach. During a pregnancy that requires bedrest, the risk pregnancy itself is a crisis that requires parents to focus their attention
and coping skills on day-to-day life. Holding a real baby in your
arms seems like a wonderful but distant dream.

While you are on bedrest, you try to shorten your sense of time
by focusing on the present day or coming days rather than on the
weeks or months ahead. Thinking about life after delivery can

make you anxious because it once again lengthens time in your mind. You can't help but notice how long this pregnancy could be, when you focus attention on your due date! The habit of not looking too far ahead is hard to break, even when it becomes realistic to think about having your baby.

Some women in high-risk pregnancy feel superstitious about making plans for the baby or recognizing their hopes for a healthy outcome. It is as though they could magically protect themselves from the pain of loss by not wanting the baby too much. But experience has shown that denying your hopeful feelings cannot protect you from disappointment and may make it harder to enjoy the baby when all goes well.

Although there are emotional difficulties in thinking about your baby's arrival, there are also benefits. Some understanding of what to expect after delivery along with good plans for support can make a great deal of difference in your adjustment to life after bedrest.

Planning for Delivery

Talk with your physician about special delivery plans for your pregnancy. Some conditions may necessitate a planned Cesarean delivery or a trial of labor with an increased probability of a C-section. Ask how your medical complication might alter your labor and delivery experience. If you are taking medication, your dose may change as you near delivery or your medication may be discontinued. Find out about medications that might be used during the delivery. If you have a cervical stitch, talk with your doctor about when the stitch will be removed.

You need to know when to call your obstetrician. In routine delivery, patients are told to call when they have a certain number of regular contractions at a specified time interval. Since your pregnancy is different, your doctor will probably have instructions specific to your situation.

The location of delivery may change depending upon the circumstances. Some obstetricians deliver in more than one hospital and may ask you to go to an alternate hospital if you are in labor early in pregnancy. If there are no hospitals in your area equipped and staffed to care for very premature or sick infants, you may be transported to a regional perinatal center if your doctor thinks that your baby will need their special help. Since hospital equipment and staffing vary, it is best if a very early or sick baby can be delivered in a facility that is prepared to offer all that is needed. This reduces the need to transport a vulnerable newborn to another hospital. It also means that mother and baby can recover in the same place.

Develop a plan for getting to the hospital. This should include emergency-care options for your other children in case you need to go quickly and unexpectedly. (If all else fails, take the children with you to the hospital and ask for help when you arrive.) Know the route to the hospital so that you can tell a neighbor how to get there if necessary. Plan alternate routes in case you need to go during heavy traffic. Some families in areas of severe winter weather line up neighbors with four-wheel-drive vehicles. Contact a number of people as backup drivers and baby-sitters so that you can be confident about getting help. Dads should be sure to leave telephone numbers as they move about during the day. Some fathers have rented paging devices so that they can be reached at all times.

You probably have a packed bag ready for the hospital trip since you know that you might go unexpectedly. The list on page 123 is a good start for packing this bag if you haven't yet done so. You need to add an outfit for your baby. You may also want your camera and a small stuffed animal to place in the bassinet.

If possible, get preadmission forms from your hospital so that much of the paperwork will be done before you arrive. Inform the labor and delivery nurses that you have been on bedrest for a period of time and explain the details of your pregnancy complication. This is another time when it helps to carry a written description of your medical history.

The Last Hours of Bedrest

As you speed along in the finishing stages of your bedrest pregnancy, you find you are pulling away from the medical complications and concentrating more on the preparations that every pregnancy requires. Imagine that pregnancy is a superhighway with exits for each week of gestation and one final finish in the delivery room. Somewhere along this route you exited the highway and have been traveling on a separate road. Amazingly, that side road has continued to parallel the highway and in fact is leading you back to the main flow of traffic. If you are near full-term delivery, much of what you experience will now be the same as any other mother.

Traveling to the hospital, you will feel the normal hopes and anxieties that every pregnant woman has on her trip to mother-hood. Aside from concern about your baby, you may be asking, "What will labor be like?" Labor and delivery seem to vary as much with bedrest mothers as they do in the general population of delivering women. Labor and delivery nurses often recommend walking in early stages of labor to help speed the process. This is helpful, but your stamina may be greatly reduced by your bedrest. Do what you can without exhausting yourself. Although your leg and abdominal muscles are weakened from bedrest, your uterus has been exercising throughout the pregnancy. You can be assured that you have at least this one toned muscle, the muscle that is most important in delivery.

One benefit of your experience is that you will enter the delivery room with more emotional flexibility than the average mother. You have adapted to so many changes throughout these many months, you won't be shocked if labor and delivery are not exactly the way you want them to be. Although you would like to have a picture-perfect birth, you have already adjusted to a less-than-perfect pregnancy. At this point, a healthy baby is your top priority. You understand that medical equipment and hospital procedures can be vital at times. You are also less likely to evaluate your mothering ability based on what you do during labor and delivery. In your efforts to maintain this pregnancy, you have already done more active mothering than you thought possible.

I spent my last hours of bedrest lying in a hospital bed, waiting for the scheduled time of my Cesarean section. As I waited, all the nurses and doctors who had seen me during my prenatal visits came in to congratulate me. They knew I was carrying a girl and I began to hear these women and men calling to each other in the hallway, "Guess what little girl is coming out tonight?" Maybe I wasn't having a standard labor and delivery, but my birth was going to be a very happy event for the hospital staff, too.

Immediately following delivery, you may have any of a number of normal reactions to the birth of your child. If there is a serious problem, you will probably be worried, sad, perhaps angry, and at the same time you could feel elated that you have made it through childbirth. Some mothers feel exhausted and emotionally numb after giving birth. They describe themselves as not quite ready to take in the reality of the baby. There is no right behavior in the delivery room. You need to do whatever is appropriate for you and your partner. You could cry, hold the baby, nurse, not hold the baby, talk, be silent, laugh, cheer, hug, babble. It is your moment. Medical personnel have seen it all, so little will surprise them. The important idea to bear in mind is that a great range of emotional reactions and expressions is normal following birth, regardless of the nature of the pregnancy.

28

*

The First Days
of Motherhood

Here you are, finally in the maternity ward, a mother. After months of separation from normal-life routines, you may be rooming with a new mother who had an uncomplicated pregnancy. If you were hospitalized prior to childbirth, you are probably transferred down the hall from high-risk antenatal to the new mothers' section. Congratulations!

For the first time, no one questions you when you get out of bed. You don't have to lie on a side or at a tilt or count the minutes that you spend sitting up or standing. And no one seems to notice this great change except you. You look like every other new mother as you walk down the hospital corridor. Like most bedrest veterans, you eagerly explore your surroundings. Even though you look like any other mother (slippers, robe, awkward walk), you may have different feelings on the inside. You could be a little dazed to be finished with your seemingly endless pregnancy and might realize that you never dared to anticipate this result.

I had three losses and over four years of effort before my child was born. I had concentrated all my energy on trying to have a baby. Now that I finally had become a mother, I felt unprepared. I had never allowed myself to make plans or daydream about holding a baby; no baby shower, no preparation of the nursery. I was scared because I had concentrated on the success of the pregnancy instead of thinking about pregnancy as just the process of becoming a mother.

Talking with your hospital nurses can help you to make the physical and emotional adjustments needed for your return to normal life. It is important to inform the maternity nurses that you have been on bedrest. Often the nursing staff who are caring for your baby are unaware that you have been on restricted activity. You need to give them this information so that they can help you cope with these immediate changes.

This is a time to tend carefully to your own body and its special needs after pregnancy bedrest. You may need to ease into the hectic schedule of the maternity ward. If you find yourself becoming exhausted after feeding the baby or walking, talk to your nurse. You may need to begin a routine of gentle exercises that can be individually designed by a physical therapist. It is not unusual for a bedrester to get additional support from health professionals after the birth of her child.

For many months you have been concentrating on all of the physiological changes in your pregnancy. Now that you are no longer pregnant, you need to direct these observation skills to your healing and recovery. Some of the physical signs that you notice will be common to most women after pregnancy; some may be specific to your medical condition. You have many experts on hand in the hospital to answer your questions and provide feedback about your progress. Talk to your doctor about what you should be experiencing and how to be alert to changes that could need prompt medical attention. Some veterans of childbirth recommend that you become familiar with the post-delivery changes in your body before you leave the hospital: you might look at your C-section incision or your episiotomy (with a mirror) so that you know exactly how it appears. That way, if you have any questions about your appearance, your doctor and nurses are available to help you.

And, since you have looked at your body, you will be able to recognize changes as you heal during the next several weeks. This familiarity could also enable you to notice a problem if one develops.

Getting to Know Your Baby

If your baby is healthy, you can spend a great deal of time together in your room becoming reacquainted in your new separate state. First-time mothers may not appreciate this service, but veteran moms are grateful for nursery care at night so that they can get some sleep. These hospital days are a good opportunity to consult with experienced nurses on baby-care issues such as bathing, cord care, bottle and breast feeding. If you do choose to breast-feed, there is no substitute for the assistance that a good breast-feeding coach can provide if she can observe how your baby is nursing.

You Are Going Home

You and your doctor will decide when you have recuperated sufficiently from delivery to continue your recovery at home. You and your baby may be discharged from the hospital on the same day, or your baby may remain in the nursery for observation and treatment during these crucial first days or weeks of life.

If Your Baby Stays in the Hospital

Leaving the hospital with empty arms is very hard to do. You need to recover from your pregnancy and, at the same time, begin long-distance parenthood. Instead of weekly trips to your doctor, you make daily trips to your baby. After weeks of restricted activity, you hop in the car, spend part of your day with your new child, and then dash around trying to handle all the other aspects of your life. If you have had a Cesarean delivery, you must also cope with recovery from major surgery. Your time with your hospitalized baby may be shortened because you are not strong enough to make frequent trips, you have other children who need your care, you have temporary driving restrictions, or the baby is in a hospital that is a long way from your home. This transition is an exhausting time for you and your family.

There are several things that other parents have found helpful in this situation:

1. Let people know what is happening to your family. Call your friends and relatives, your church or synagogue, your support group, your neighbors. As much as you care to, share what you know about your baby's condition and your feelings and support needs. Don't hide your pain or worry.

2. Get information. Find out how to contact the nursery before you leave the hospital. What hours can you call? Can you call in the middle of the night if you want to check on your child? Is there a primary nurse for your child?

3. Learn about your baby's condition. Find out what to expect— the typical ups and downs for infants like this. Talk to the neonatologist, find books on the condition, ask the hospital social worker if there is a support group for this complication in your community. Learn about the equipment, tests, and treatments that are likely to be used to help your baby. An excellent resource book for parents of premature babies is *The Premature Baby Book* by Helen Harrison (St. Martin's Press, New York, 1983).

4. Take care of yourself. Recognize that you need a lot of rest, good food, and a great deal of support.

5. Use the teamwork skills that you and the baby's father developed during pregnancy. Do the things that you did before to help each other. Try to share your feelings. In addition to your mutual support, you will both need a chance to lean on people who are not as upset as the two of you.

6. Continue to accept help. Give family and friends specific tasks, such as cooking, shopping, cleaning a bathroom, giving you a ride to the hospital, taking care of other children.

7. Learn how you can be an active parent when you visit your baby in the nursery. Remember that this is *your* baby. You can talk,

sing, touch, and perhaps feed and hold your child. The doctors and nurses are there to lend their expertise, but you decide what treatments you will accept for your child.

When Your Baby Comes Home

Whether your baby's homecoming is immediate or delayed, the moment you strap him into the car seat, you mark the end of one phase of your life and a new beginning for your family. What a day this is! Many high-risk parents are stunned at their good fortune when they leave the hospital with a healthy newborn. You may be surprised if you have spent the previous months anticipating a premature baby. It can be such a thrill to leave the hospital in the company of your new child, perhaps the first thing you've done in this pregnancy that felt normal. Welcome to the world of parenthood!

The car seat that we mention is as important to your baby as all of the high-tech medicine that went into his arrival. It's hard to resist the temptation to cradle your child in your arms as you ride, but a child's life is too precious to risk. If you don't own a car seat, ask the hospital staff about car-seat lending programs in your community. If your baby is very small or has breathing problems, be sure to consult with the neonatologist about positioning your child and choosing a car seat design that is appropriate for a premature infant.

If your baby stayed in the hospital longer than you did, her homecoming can be both joyous and anxious:

My daughter spent sixteen days in the neonatal intensive care nursery with specialized nurses providing twenty-four-hour attention to her every breath, heartbeat, and temperature fluctuation. As we neared the time when she would come home, I began to wonder how I could possibly take care of such a fragile baby. When the moment finally arrived to take her home, it was obvious that she needed a diaper change. "Here, you do it," said the nurse. My self-doubts mushroomed as I realized I wasn't even sure how to change a diaper! It took a few weeks of mothering to realize that my daughter no longer needed the twenty-four-hour care of those professional nurses—she needed me.

If Your Baby Never Comes Home

It feels awful to think about losing a baby, but most parents wonder about this possibility, especially when a pregnancy is labeled high-risk. Perhaps the most important thing to do if your baby dies is to allow the natural healing process of grief to take place. The pain can feel unbearable, but all of us have the capacity to grieve and heal given the time, space, and support that we need. Please see Appendix 2, "Pregnancy Loss," for advice from bereaved parents.

Coping Strategies for the Bedrest Veteran

After you've heard the umpteenth remark about being well rested for motherhood, you may begin to wonder if you really do have the strength to make it through the first weeks at home. Don't discard all of your good pregnancy bedrest skills just because you are able to run around. Instead, use the experience of the last few months to help you cope with the days ahead. You know how to get simple, nutritious meals, limit housework, and screen visitors. You can delegate jobs and coordinate volunteers.

Help is essential. A mother and newborn can manage all alone, but not without great distress. It is tempting for women who have needed a lot of assistance to dismiss their helpers the minute the baby arrives. Don't make this mistake! Exhaustion is a high price to pay for independence.

Fatigue is the most common complaint for postpartum parents. It is crucial that this be taken seriously and limited as much as possible. Ongoing sleep deprivation, when there is no relief in sight, can too easily lead to depression. What should you do when you feel tired? This is a time to look at your days and nights to see where you could get more rest. Are you so eager to be back to normal that you are doing too much and accepting too little help?

Are you letting yourself nap when the baby sleeps? Some mothers feel lazy when they sleep during the day, not realizing that napping is essential when nights are disturbed. Do you stay awake to take care of your other young children? Think about finding someone who can come over to watch all of your children, including the baby, so that you can count on having a regular nap each day until you feel more rested. With someone else listening for the baby, you may find that you can drift into a deeper sleep.

What About My Body?

You will feel weak and find that you have lost some muscle tone. Your general endurance (cardiovascular fitness) will be less than it was before your pregnancy. The good news is that some of your strength and energy returns within a week or so as you once again get comfortable standing and walking. With your doctor's help, you can design a very gradual exercise program to help you recover. Walking and swimming are terrific forms of exercise, easily adaptable to your changing fitness level. It is crucial that you proceed slowly and support your health program with good nutrition and as much rest as you can possibly get with a new baby.

29

*

It's All Over—
or Is It?

If your baby is born healthy, the time of risk is ended and your
stressful situation is all over—or is it? Many mothers and fathers
find themselves in a curious position following a healthy delivery.
Friends and family who have been faithful in their support are
celebrating the birth with exuberance. They can put a complete
and satisfying close to the stressful experience of bedrest and
rejoice without reservation. For the parents who are not quite
ready or able to forget, it can be painful to compare their own
feelings with those of their family and friends.

"What's wrong with me?" a new mother asks. "I feel so tense
and I'm just not that close to the baby. Maybe I can't bond!" With
all the media emphasis on bonding, parents can begin to panic if
they aren't filled with deep feelings of love right from the start. In
reality, it is not unusual for a new parent to feel a bit detached from
a baby even after a routine pregnancy.

A medically risky pregnancy involves emotional tasks that
greatly complicate the bonding process after birth. During your
pregnancy you had to prepare to accept a new child while you also

prepared for the possibility that the new child might not live. This brings about a kind of grieving throughout the pregnancy that doesn't automatically end at delivery. A tremendous amount of emotional energy has gone into coping with the stress brought about by the serious complications of your pregnancy. It is as though you were running a marathon and suddenly had to sit down for tea and cakes at the finish line. Try as you might, you can't help sweating, panting, and being preoccupied with the race.

You could also compare yourself to a soldier who has been in combat. In the midst of battle, a soldier must be alert to the events around him. If he pays attention to personal feelings, he takes his mind from the battle and risks disaster. As long as the war lasts, there is little escape from danger. Often the emotional impact of combat does not emerge until the war is over and it is safe to relax. Of course, a high-risk pregnancy is not a battle situation, but it does have similar characteristics: chronic stress and the question of survival.

Ann delivered a healthy daughter after fifteen weeks of bedrest including ten weeks in the hospital:

I returned home four days after Sarah's birth. My husband was overcome with joy to have us together again and continually said, "It's so wonderful to have you home." I was touched by his happiness but confused by my own feelings. I didn't really know where I was. I couldn't seem to bridge the gap between the otherworldliness of institutional life and the home life I had left several months previously.

During the weeks following Sarah's birth, it was difficult for me to grasp that her safe arrival was a reality. I continued to awaken each morning with a terror in my heart that a bleed might strike and jeopardize her life. I would then realize that the danger no longer existed—that Sarah was safe and healthy. It took months for me to experience my body as my own. Slowly I learned not to dread a sneeze and not to censor an urge to bend down and pick something up. A thousand times a day I became aware, as if for the first time, that the pregnancy was *over.* As I gradually developed

my awareness of Sarah's safe arrival, many of my unex-
pressed emotions began to emerge. I walked around for
months with tears streaming from my eyes. I felt enormous
relief tinged with wonder.

It may be difficult to say good-bye to your doctors and nurses
after your battle is over and you return to postpartum peacetime.
During these weeks you have developed a special relationship with
your health professional support team. They were an intimate part
of your life. You got to know them just as you were being cut off
from all the contacts of a normal pregnancy. They were the people
to whom you complained, who comforted you when you cried, and
who cheered you in your success. Now they have turned their
efforts to the next bedrest patients. You have become one of many
postpartum patients who return for routine checkups, bringing
dozens of pictures of newborns, toddlers, and big kids. Maybe you
feel a little abandoned. Some mothers find it helpful to schedule a
follow-up appointment that allows enough time to review the
events of the pregnancy and ask questions about the future. Aside
from medical concerns, there are many feelings you may want to
share after this intense experience.

You can take heart knowing that you and your child will always
be special, no matter how many dramatic pregnancies are handled
by this team. Most medical professionals love to see the pictures
and want to know how you are. Their advice to keep in touch is not
meant lightly. The recovery from a medically complicated pregnancy may progress more slowly than routine recovery. You may
have more than one postpartum office visit during the first few
months after childbirth.

What Is Normal Now?

If you are trying to decide if you are "back to normal," don't make
the mistake of looking back to life before baby for comparison. You
have a new peer group now composed of all the countless new
parents in the world. No new parents could really be called normal.
As normal as parenthood may be, the transition to the job is far

from routine. Even women with fantastic pregnancies and glowing delivery-room experiences will tell you that these early days are tiring, complicated, chaotic, and emotional. You may experience the baby blues. This short-lived and common response to birth can include sadness, anxiety, crying spells, forgetfulness, fatigue, and irritability. Luckily, these hormone storms are brief and usually go away on their own. (Postpartum depression is described in Appendix 1.)

Becoming a parent is a series of adjustments that seems awkward at first, but becomes more natural with practice. Before you draw the conclusion that all your new feelings are related to the kind of pregnancy that you had, compare notes with the mothers around you to get a sense of normal life for new moms.

Will I Ever Get Over My Bedrest Experience?

Many women immersed in the high stress of a high-risk pregnancy begin to wonder if they will be able to cope after the baby is born. After receiving bad news more than once in a pregnancy, you can become pessimistic about a lot of things. One mother told us that she just assumed she would have a postpartum depression since everything else had gone wrong in her pregnancy. Fortunately, her dire prediction was wrong.

What we can say from experience with many high-risk mothers is that there is a great variety of emotional responses to delivery. Having a risk pregnancy means that you've been under stress, but it does not mean that you will automatically have depressed feelings after the birth. Your emotional recovery will be different from the average, but the coping skills you have been developing throughout the pregnancy will be there to support you.

It may help to think in terms of recovery-time differences rather than using the label "depression." Your body will naturally need more time to return to normal than the body of a mother who was on her feet for nine months. Those leg muscles will strengthen with use. In the same way, your feelings will take more time to recover than those of a woman who was low-risk. You had to prepare for things to go badly, to ready yourself to cope if you had to leave the hospital empty-handed. This took emotional energy. You reached deep into your reserves to find the strength to cope. Now it will take some time to replenish those reserves. For most parents, time, support, and the opportunity to talk are all that are needed to recover from this event in their lives.

You can help to end this chapter of your life by telling others about it. Friends and family may be supportive, but eventually will get a bit tired of hearing the stories. Try to notice when others have heard enough and seek another listener. Some people will have trouble understanding why you want to talk and will say, "It's all over! Stop thinking about it." Although they mean well, they don't recognize that it is not all over for you and that, by talking, you are slowly recovering so that you can go on to something new.

Support groups can be terrific when you need to talk. Some mothers find good help in a new mothers' group, even though they may be the only high-risk pregnancy in the group. Others feel too frustrated comparing their experiences with someone else's complaints about a routine pregnancy. If this is how you feel, seek out others who have had risk pregnancies, too. Reliving and sharing your experiences with other bedrest veterans can be helpful in the process of emotional recovery. Some women have formed informal groups; other groups are facilitated by a therapist. Sharing your memories with other women who really understand what you felt makes it easier to express fears you never allowed yourself to feel during your pregnancy.

Sometimes support groups don't seem to be enough and you may want to consider talking to a therapist who is skilled in pregnancy-related concerns. Seeking this support is not a failure, but a positive, strong step toward healing.

Ellen spent four months on bedrest hoping to prevent the premature birth of her second child. Her first child was born at thirty-two weeks. When Ellen delivered a healthy daughter, she was surprised to find that her feelings of being at risk lingered. Like many veteran bedresters, she was waiting for the other shoe to drop. She also found herself dwelling on disturbing memories from the pregnancy. Her story is not unusual:

At thirty-seven weeks my baby was born, a healthy, six-pound girl. Now I could go back to a normal life, I had thought. But I found that it was not easy to put the experience of my pregnancy behind me. . . .

My months in bed had been traumatic. . . . I continued to find it hard not to expect something terrible to happen. It seemed that I had been emotionally braced for crisis for so long that I could not believe that everything was finally okay. It was impossible to instantly shift gears into a non-crisis mentality.

I had felt deeply hurt by a lack of support, both emotional and logistical, from relatives and friends during my pregnancy. Afterward, I continued to dwell in my thoughts on how let down I had been by everyone's reaction. Many people had treated my situation so lightly and my impression had been that they thought I was just relaxing in bed, not actively fighting for my baby's life and health. I was constantly assured that everything would be fine. While I wanted to maintain a positive attitude, I also needed to be realistic about the seriousness of my condition. I knew I had no guarantees that even if I did everything my doctors told me to do, my baby would be full-term and healthy. But few people had been able to provide support for me to talk about my fears. For the most part, I kept them bottled up inside as I concentrated all my emotional strength on just getting through the pregnancy.

After my daughter's birth, it all seemed to come to the surface. I felt depressed and seemed to have no emotional stamina to deal with everyday problems and stresses. . . . My pregnancy continued to affect me. Yet it was hard to find support at that point, too. After all, everything had turned out perfectly. At times, I wondered if I was overreacting, that perhaps the situation had not been as serious as I had felt it to be. For me, the solution lay in therapy. After time with an understanding therapist and much reflection, I was able to come to terms with what had happened and my reaction to it. I gradually came to realize that my fears had been justified and that my feelings after my pregnancy made sense. The fear of losing my baby was a very powerful emotion for me and I could not treat it lightly. It was not wrong to feel depressed even after a happy resolution; in fact, it was necessary for me to experience these feelings in order to work through my experience and move on.

As I now look back on my pregnancy two years later, I can see many positive results (in addition to a wonderful daughter!). I am proud of myself, my husband, and son for how we endured what, for us, was a really tough time. I have no doubt that we're stronger for it . . . I think I'll always envy women who have carefree and active pregnancies, for whom the expectation of a healthy, full-term baby is never in question. But I've come to believe that our experience has given us a different perspective than we might have otherwise had. Building our family has been difficult, but perhaps that has made us all the more precious to each other.

You won't get over your bedrest in the sense that you will ever forget about it, but you will discover that you gradually think less often of the past, and the feelings that come when you do remember pregnancy are not as intense. It is important to recognize what hard work you have been doing during this pregnancy; you need time to adjust to a nonrisk life.

For many of you, the recognition of your passage to normal parenthood will come in a scene like the following when you catch yourself sharing positive memories of your pregnancy.

I was introduced to my cousin's close friend who had heard tales of my unusual pregnancy throughout the time that I was in bed. She was fascinated with the medical complications that she had heard about and seemed eager to hear all the details of my trouble. She said, "Wasn't it unbearable to stay in bed so long and wonder when your blood pressure would shoot up again?" I said, "It was hard, but look at this beautiful baby!" Then I started to tell some of the funny

things that happened when I couldn't get up. We all laughed
so much. I was delighted to realize that I finally declined an
invitation to tell my war stories.

When It's Time to Put This Book Away

When you were first given this book, you might have clutched it
like a life preserver. Now it lies among all the baby-care books,
reminding you of a worn stuffed animal that you outgrew.

It's good to outgrow things. Some of the items that your children will outgrow may be given to others, but certain books, toys,
and baby clothes will remain in your attic for you to share with your
children and grandchildren.

We can't predict how pregnancy complications will be treated
when all of our children are young adults beginning their families.
We hope that this book will be part of the memories you will share
with the next generation about the "good old days" when you
became a mother.

APPENDICES

APPENDIX 1

*

Postpartum Depression

Will I Have Postpartum Depression Because of My Bedrest?

The good news is that serious postpartum depression is an unusual phenomenon. Hormones and genetic predisposition may play as big a role in this type of depression as situational factors such as marital problems, lack of support, role adjustment, and stressful pregnancy.

Does high-risk pregnancy make you more likely to be seriously depressed after delivery? The research in this area is limited and the results are mixed. In a review of studies on postpartum depression, authors Michael W. O'Hara and Ellen M. Zekoski report "data regarding the relation between obstetrical complications and postpartum depression are puzzling. Several studies have found a significant positive association and several studies have found a significant negative association" ("Postpartum Depression: A Comprehensive Review," *Motherhood and Mental Illness, Vol. 2: Causes and Consequences*, I. F. Brockington and R. Kumar, eds. [London: Wright, 1988], pp. 17–63).

For a small number of new parents, the support of family, friends, and peer groups will not be enough to help them get back to normal. They may show signs of serious difficulty, such as appetite changes leading to large weight loss or gain; trouble sleeping (when there is an opportunity to sleep); preoccupation with disturbing thoughts; agitation; chronic feelings of sadness, worthlessness, and guilt; self-destructive thoughts; or extreme difficulty in establishing closeness with the baby. If you, your partner, or other child experience any of these symptoms, it may be wise to consult a mental health professional who has experience with new parents. You can ask the professionals who have been involved in your pregnancy or the local mental health association for a referral.

APPENDIX 2

*

Pregnancy Loss

The death of your child is such a painful experience. In the first days of grief, you wonder if you can ever recover from your loss. Parents who have lost babies advise others who are bereaved to do these things:

1. Make your baby's existence as real as possible. It is easier to say good-bye when we affirm that the child once lived (if only in the womb).
2. Name the baby. This helps confirm the fact that you lost a real child.
3. See the baby. This may scare you, but what you imagine is probably worse than how your baby actually looks. Don't be afraid that seeing your deceased child will make grieving harder. Long after a loss, parents who avoided seeing the baby often wish that they had looked at their child.
4. Ask to hold the baby. You have a right to do this if you want. You should have and take as much time with your child as you feel you need. This is important, and while it may be difficult to do at this point, you will be very grateful in the future that you have done it.

5. Create mementos by taking pictures, cutting a lock of hair. (Many hospitals routinely photograph babies who die and have pictures available for parents to see at a later date.)

6. Make a memory book or box in which to keep hospital records, wrist band, blanket, footprints, pictures.

7. Consider having a funeral or memorial service to share your grief with others.

8. Seek support from your religious beliefs and members of the clergy. Rabbis, priests, and ministers are available to you whether or not you attend religious services.

9. Plant a tree or flowers, make a donation to charity in your baby's name.

10. Join a support group for people who have lost a baby. The Compassionate Friends, Inc., is a national organization for bereaved parents that can provide referrals to groups in your area. The address of their national headquarters is: P.O. Box 1347, Oak Brook, IL 60521; phone (312) 323-5010.

11. Read books about pregnancy loss and grief.

12. Seek professional help from a perinatal bereavement specialist if you feel that you need more than family and community support. Be sure you go as a couple to the initial sessions, since grief is a family problem no matter who shows the most symptoms.

Following some of the above suggestions may not be possible when the loss is an early fetal death. Other suggestions you may not choose to do. There is no right way to grieve. What is most important is to trust your instincts and find people who can support you as you heal in your own unique way.

With the exception of rather unusual circumstances, it is highly unlikely that you did anything that caused or contributed to the death of your child. It is normal and natural to always seek a reason when tragedy occurs, but in so doing, be sure that you are not inappropriately pointing the finger at yourself. Your partner is also grieving, may feel guilt, and could be secretly wondering if you did something that contributed to the loss. These thoughts are very hard to say out loud, even though they are common and natural. If the two of you grieve at a different pace or intensity, you can become very upset with each other. Try very hard to talk about your loss and all of the strong feelings that you are having. Couples who avoid sharing their grief may have lasting relationship problems as a result.

Be prepared for some friends, family members, and acquaintances to avoid you, become very awkward around you, or say hurtful things such as, "You're young, you can have another one." Most people mean well but fail to realize that your baby was a real child to you. In their minds, you lost a "potential" child. People can become anxious about the intensity of your grief and give you subtle cues that perhaps you should be finished now. They don't understand the healing power of grief.

Feel free to discuss your feelings and concerns with your health-care provider or, as many do, seek counseling to help you through what is at best a most difficult time. Have faith in yourselves and your ability to heal.

APPENDIX 3

＊

Checklist: What Does Bedrest Mean for Me?

This chart was developed by Lenette Moses of Intensive Caring Unlimited, a Philadelphia/Southern New Jersey parent support group. Please address questions and comments to Lenette Moses, ICU, 910 Bent Lane, Philadelphia, PA 19118.

What Can I Do Right Now?	*Date*	*Week of Pregnancy*
1. Activity Level		
maintain a normal activity level	————	————
slightly decrease activity level	————	————
greatly decrease activity level	————	————
2. Working Outside the Home		
maintain my full-time job	————	————
work part-time (number of hours?)	————	————
work in my home (how many hours?)	————	————
stop work completely	————	————
why: ———————————————————————		

	Date	Week of Pregnancy

3. Working Inside the Home
continue doing all housework   _____   _____
decrease housework
   (laundry? heavy cleaning?)   _____   _____
preparing meals (standing up)   _____   _____
vigorous scrubbing   _____   _____
other: _____
why: _____

4. Child Care
care for other children as usual   _____   _____
no lifting   _____   _____
active toddler needs caretaker   _____   _____
full-time caretaker needed for children   _____   _____
why: _____

5. Driving
may drive car as usual   _____   _____
passenger only   _____   _____
car rides only to doctor or medical test   _____   _____
why: _____

6. Lying-Down Time (restrictions)
continue normal standing, and sitting   _____   _____
sit down frequently (limited mobility)   _____   _____
lie down during day (how many hours?)   _____   _____
side-lying all day (describe position)   _____   _____
side-lying with hips tilted all day   _____   _____
climb stairs (how many times each day?)   _____   _____
no climbing stairs   _____   _____
why: _____

7. Mealtimes
lying down   _____   _____
sitting up (for how long?)   _____   _____

	Date	Week of Pregnancy
sitting at table	____	____

why: _____

8. Bathroom Privileges

	Date	Week of Pregnancy
may go to bathroom as usual	____	____
need bedpan or commode at bedside	____	____
may take shower (how often? how long?)	____	____
may take tub baths (how often? how long?)	____	____
wash hair in shower?	____	____
wash hair sitting in shower?	____	____
hair can be washed while lying down	____	____

why: _____

9. Sexual Relations

	Date	Week of Pregnancy
continue normal sexual relations	____	____
limit certain activities	____	____
avoid sexual activities leading to female orgasm	____	____
avoid sexual intercourse	____	____

why: _____

10. Pregnancy Monitoring

	Date	Week of Pregnancy
monitor fetal movements (need specific instructions)	____	____
home monitoring equipment (need specific instructions)	____	____

should take (drug) _____

__times daily, dosage: _____

side effects: _____

why: _____

medical tests and procedures:

	Date	Week of Pregnancy
amniocentesis	____	____

	Date	Week of Pregnancy
sonograms	_____	_____
blood sugar screening	_____	_____
nonstress tests	_____	_____
stress tests	_____	_____
other blood tests: _____		
why: _____		
stop cigarette smoking	_____	_____
why: _____		
follow these dietary rules	_____	_____
plenty of: _____		
avoid: _____		
why: _____		

11. My Health Care Team

	Name	Phone no.
OB/GYN doctor(s)	_____	_____
nurse(s)	_____	_____
physical therapist	_____	_____
occupational therapist	_____	_____
social worker	_____	_____
dietitian	_____	_____

If Problems Arise

When should I contact my doctor? _____

Where will I be hospitalized? _____

Where might I be transferred? _____

Name of OB/GYN at other hospital? _____

Where would my baby be hospitalized? _____

Could the father be present at
    delivery? _____

Is there a possibility of Cesarean
    surgery? _____

APPENDIX 4

✳

Checklist: Hospital to Home

1. What can I take home from the hospital?
   _____
   _____
   _____

2. My doctor _____
   telephone _____

3. My nurse _____
   telephone _____

4. My physical therapist _____
   telephone _____
   exercises (on separate sheet) _____

5. My occupational therapist _____
   telephone _____

6. My dietitian _____
   telephone _____
   diet plan (on separate sheet) _____

7. My social worker _____
   telephone _____

8. How am I getting home from the hospital?
   driver: _____
   time: _____

9. Follow-up telephone call after I get home:
   person: _____
   telephone: __ _____
   time to call back: _____

10. My Next Appointment: date: _____
                                time: _____
                                place: _____

11. My special warning signals:

    _____
    _____
    _____
    _____

12. How do I get back into the hospital quickly?
    PLAN A _____

    _____
    PLAN B _____

    _____

ACKNOWLEDGMENTS

✳

This book is a revision and expansion of the 1986 book we published privately. We wish to thank the nurses, doctors, social workers, physical therapists, occupational therapists, and pregnancy bedresters who used that first version and encouraged us with their letters. Their enthusiastic response demonstrated the need for a special book focused on the nonmedical issues of pregnancy bedrest.

There are many physicians who provided excellent suggestions for this book: David A. Nagey, M.D., Ph.D.; John J. Schruefer, M.D.; Luis Sanz, M.D.; Elizabeth Herz, M.D.; Jeffrey C. King, M.D.; Joseph Collea, M.D.; and Allen Sandler, M.D.

We wish to thank the nurses who provided valuable contributions to the expansion of the book: Rae K. Grad, R.N., Ph.D., Executive Director, National Commission to Prevent Infant Mortality; Mary Lou Moore, Ph.D., R.N.C., A.C.C.E., F.A.A.N.; Bowman Gray School of Medicine; Judith Nierenberg, M.A., R.N., Director of Educational Resources, *American Journal of Nursing*; Pamela Pitman, R.N., B.S.N., Beloit Memorial Hospital; Connie Henry, R.N., Arlington Hospital; Tammy Arbeter, R.N.C., Pennsylvania Hospital; Judith Gunderson, R.N., B.S.N., A.C.C.E., Brigham and Women's Hospital; Dee Young, R.N., Modesto Arts Medical Group; Pam Rillstone, R.N.C., M.S.N.,

Baptist Memorial Center; Gail Greenfield, R.N., B.S.N.; Artie Achterkirch, N.P., Mork Women's Clinic; Ann Reinhardt, R.N.; Leith Mullaly, R.N., M.S.N., The Alexandria Hospital; and L.C.D.R.s Mary Ann Baumann, N.C., U.S.N., and Marianne Frank, N.C., U.S.N., who contributed to the book during their personal time.

Jane Frahm, P.T., Hutzel Hospital; Judy Giergielewicz, R.P.T., Mercy Medical Center; and Diane Peeso, R.N., Lutheran Hospital–LaCrosse, provided important information about the most current advances in physical therapy protocols for antepartum patients. Jane Frahm is also thanked for introducing two new phrases to the pregnancy bedrester vocabulary: side-lying and gravity-sensitive pregnancy complications.

Jane Richman, M.S.W., Infant Care Program, Evanston Hospital, contributed many ideas for our chapters on hospitalization. Sharon Covington, M.S.W., provided advice on issues concerning pregnancy loss. Beverlee Heinztelman, M.S.W., the Children's Hospital National Medical Center, contributed to our earlier drafts.

The Confinement Line volunteers are thanked for their help. The Childbirth Education Association, Inc., of northern Virginia is also thanked for its continued sponsorship of this nonprofit support network and the encouragement of this book.

Intensive Caring Unlimited, a nonprofit parent support group program serving metropolitan Philadelphia and southern New Jersey, has been outstanding in its support as our manuscript evolved. Lynette Moses, the newsletter editor, is thanked for her wonderful bedrest checklist, which appears in the Appendices.

Dr. Michael W. O'Hara, Ph.D., is thanked for providing information and insights for Appendix 1, "Postpartum Depression."

R. Michael Wilson, Cheryl Hammer, Roberta Peyser, and Beatrice Avick were instrumental in providing initial suggestions for the revision of the chapters. Judy Howard gave her excellent proofreading skills between nursing sessions with baby Hannah. Jack Sauer and Pam Marvin continued to believe in the importance of supporting women on bedrest.

Sara Larson edited our 1986 book and returned to edit our

expansion of the chapters. Then and now, she provided cogent and constructive criticism. She melded our writing styles into one book with two strong voices. Her insight, as a mother of three, was invaluable in identifying issues we needed to address. Above all, she was patient and persistent with each of us, steadily honing our chapters until only the quality work remained.

Cynthia Vartan, our book editor, has provided us with the confidence to pursue our ideas for the expansion of the book. Her consistent words of encouragement were very much appreciated.

Sarah Freymann, of Stepping Stone Literary Agency, saw the potential of our book and was its advocate. She provided us with excellent suggestions for expanding our original version. Her advice to focus on a bedrester's perception of time throughout a high-risk pregnancy was a valuable contribution.

Moses L. Jackson, our illustrator, managed to transform our many ideas into four beautiful pictures for this book. We wanted pictures of bedresters successfully managing the nuts and bolts of daily tasks. We gave him our stick-figure drawings and our draft chapters. He figured out what we really needed and drew and redrew each picture until it had all the right props and the correct angles for side-lying and hip elevation. He has done more than illustrate our ideas—he has created positive images.

We thank Sue's brother, David Holyoke, who was her guide through the world of word-processing. Deborah's husband, Alan, continued to give unstintingly of his software, terminal, and printer, through each stage of the manuscript's production.

We would like to thank the many pregnancy bedresters and their families whose stories enrich our text. Their ideas and experiences provide perspectives much needed by readers. The humorous and disheartening moments of their high-risk pregnancies are a valuable contribution to understanding the realities of bedrest.

It has not been easy to spend coffee breaks, lunches, and evenings listening to a colleague's frustration with faxes and word processors. We thank our colleagues at Potomac Psychological Resources and the Personnel Department of the National Naval Medical Center for their patience and tolerance.

We thank David Park of Giant Printing in Arlington, Virginia, for his technical advice and prompt service in printing our original version of this book.

We would also like to thank Ann McCoy and Margaret Barnett of the U.S. Postal Service and Gary Ross of Mail Boxes, Etc., who have helped us send our manuscript drafts and books to health professionals and bedresters.

Our families have been created through the anguish and turmoil of high-risk pregnancies. For our husbands and children, life with our bedrest pregnancies has been followed by life with our helping others manage their pregnancy bedrests. Our love for our family members has been the driving force to help other expectant parents. We both liked what we wrote to each of our families four years ago and would like to repeat it here:

Susan thanks her first child, daughter Kylie, who taught her what a miracle a baby's life can be. Her son, Ryan, who survived it all, makes the hard work seem well worth it. Rick, her husband and partner in life, learned the danger of serving soggy cereal, and kept on giving even when it hurt. She thanks him most of all.

Deborah is proud to the point of inarticulateness of her daughter, Julia Rose. When Julia reads this book, she will have no trouble identifying stories about the expectant parents who became her mother and father. It is hoped that she will recognize that she is the embodiment of their dreams. Alan endured sinkfuls of dirty dishes, haphazard meals, and dusty floors, indulging the specious argument that all this would make his wife a better writer. He always believed that they would become parents and that this would become a book, and for this belief, he is loved and trusted.

February 1990

ABOUT THE AUTHORS

✳

Susan Holyoke Johnston, M.S.W., is a Board Certified Diplomate in Clinical Social Work. She is a licensed clinical social worker and psychotherapist in private practice in northern Virginia. She founded The Confinement Line, a telephone support network for women on pregnancy bedrest, serving women in the Washington, D.C., metropolitan area. She leads high-risk pregnancy support groups and consults on perinatal mental health concerns.

Susan lives with her husband, Rick, daughter, Kylie, son, Ryan, a dog, and a cat in a chronically renovated old house in McLean, Virginia.

Deborah Aviva Kraut, a specialist in personnel management, focusing on job analysis and classification of medical occupations, works at the Naval Hospital of the National Naval Medical Center in Bethesda, Maryland. She holds a master's degree in industrial and labor relations (M.I.L.R.) from Cornell University and a master of education degree (M.Ed.) from The American University in Washington, D.C. She has previously authored a monograph on supportive services for disadvantaged workers, published by the New York State School for Industrial and Labor Relations in 1973. She was the director of the 1979 Summer Jobs for Youth Program co-sponsored by the Greater Washington Board of Trade and the National Alliance of Business. She frequently lectures to continuing education groups in nursing on the nonmedical issues of pregnancy bedrest. Deborah, her husband, Alan, her daughter, Julia Rose, and Deborah's bedrest foam bolster, "Jaws," live in Bethesda, Maryland.

INDEX

*

261

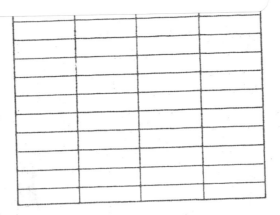